Running Wild And Running Free

By Alan S Watts

To Brooke,
Run Wild, Run free,
Run for your dreams
They're closer than they
seem.
All the Best,
Alan Watts

Running Wild And Running Free
ISBN: 978 – 1 -8380631 – 0 – 8

First published in Great Britain
in 2020 through Ingram Spark
self-publishing service

Produced by samanthahoughton.co.uk

Dedication

This book is dedicated to my children - my cheeky monkey and my little toad.

My parents and my sister and to those lifelong friends who have been part of my life through the good, the bad and the ugly times.

To my Godmother for inspiring me without realising.

Contents

Acknowledgements

Thank you to Sam Houghton for her encouragement and mentoring along my writing journey.

Thank you to the coaches who have assisted me along my Journey - Ivan Vickers, Debbie Huxton, Luke Scott III, Eugina O Liberty, Sia Di, Jay Diamond, Manny Wolfe, Tony & Nikki Vee, Jeffrey Lestz, Bob Safford Jnr, Steve Jenkins, Jacqui Rodgers, Chuck Schultz and Julie Keywell.

Thank you for your Music - Iron Maiden, Metallica, Mike Tramp and Pete Friesen.

Foreword

Wow, it's great. I love the descriptions of the emotions that some of us clearly find confusing and lock away as to being our own fault or battle. Your explanations of how if we perceive them differently has a totally different outcome on our own mental health.

Well done on your whole journey, I think by people reading this they will soon relate to it, if not the same exact experiences physically, then emotionally. Changing your outlook certainly has made a massive impact!

Dawn Fulford – Reiki Practitioner

Prologue

Arriving home from my friend's house, unaware that it was a homecoming that I would never forget for the rest of my life, let alone the impact it would have on me.

After a hard day's play, my friend Philip's mum dropped me at my front door, it was very quiet once I got inside, and as an excited six-year-old, I ran through the house full of beans. I got to the front room and saw what was in front of me, which caught me completely by surprise. My dad was lying on the sofa with my sister, both crying. I'd seen my sister cry no end - but dad? No, this was new to me, he was big and strong. I couldn't help but wonder what could make him cry. He was brought up in an age where naughty boys got the cane at school; whatever that was, it sounded worse than standing by the headmaster's office door. Boys and men were not supposed to cry. I was so confused, my heart speeded up and slowed down for no reason and I felt like my energy had vanished; I just didn't get it.

I have written this book as I believe there are some things in this world not often talked about. How little things in childhood can have a massive impact in adult years as well as opening up and sharing many things I have often felt too trapped inside myself to let out. My journey through life from being blissfully unaware that I had no connection with my feelings the majority of the time, living in places of internal anger, frustration and depression without knowing I was there. Having some amazing experiences growing up but not knowing at the time they were amazing, with great lessons hidden within those times. Looking for the world around me to change to the way I thought it should be. The disconnection from myself and my emotions lead me to have some difficulties in building relationships with the opposite sex.

So why now? Because now I feel free in a way that I never believed was possible, and in sharing this journey to get to where I am today, I aim to inspire other people to open up and share the world inside which may have been locked away for years.

1

Can This Boy Speak?

Forget Batman, Superman and all of the others, although they had some pretty cool tricks they were not my hero's. My dad was my hero and my dream for myself was to be just like him. Not just to be like him but to follow in his footsteps and take on the family farm when I grew up; there was nothing else for me! Anytime someone would ask me what I wanted to be when I grew up, my answer was always the same. *"To be a farmer like my dad."*

If my mum was there, she would often say after, *"He is also going to be a mechanic as well so he has something to fall back on."* To be fair, I was often more interested in tractors than the animals.

Growing up, out in the sticks, had its good points and bad points. Living far away from people it was harder to make friends and those friends we did have, were often other farmers' kids. There was a strong sense of community with farmers, often those with teenage children would get them babysitting for other farmers' kids. The farmers' kids would all play together while the parents talked about grown-up stuff, though we all had something in common to start from. We would often get to help feed lambs and calves, and watch them grow up, though it was never like they were pets, and it was very different from having a dog or a cat.

The farm was started by my grandparents on dad's side, their two sons, dad and my uncle worked on the farm and in my early years. There were three or four staff also, a total of three farmhouses, 400 cattle and 300 sheep. There were 4 of us kids on the farm, my 2 cousins, myself, and my sister. Traditionally farms were passed down from father to son. My mum also grew up on a farm about ten miles away, she was one of six children, one boy and five girls, sadly the first-born daughter died as a baby. My mum was the eldest of the other five.

I often told my parents that I needed glasses, which may have been more because dad wore glasses than because I couldn't see. Eventually, they took me to see the optician to be tested but we were told I didn't need them. I was gutted and my desires to be just like my dad didn't end there. Sunday lunch was always a family get together, often spent with grandparents on either side. Some things were almost guaranteed to happen; before lunch, they would all have a glass of sherry, maybe two. At one point dad noticed that the level of the sweet sherry was going down from Sunday to Sunday without dad having any in between.

So, one-week dad asked me if I wanted to try some, I said, *"Yes please,"* and drank the whole glass. A very cheeky way of finding out which child was guilty! Though what you may not expect is that he would have his sherry in a wine glass not a sherry glass. It made me a little sick that day, but it put me off alcohol for years!

I spent less time on the farm when I was of age to go to nursery school. It was fun at times, but it took me a while to settle in, though it was useful that I had one or two farm friends there as well as my cousins and sister.

The first year of junior school was the year things started to significantly change for me, my new teacher was very strict and more than a little intimidating. To me, she felt like a cross between Margaret Thatcher and the Wicked Witch of the West. To say she scared me to death would be an understatement, but at least I got to sit next to my friend Philip, which was a little comfort. It was very different from nursery school where the teacher was much younger, prettier, and very friendly. I didn't like school from that moment on, I hated it; well the lessons anyway. During the break time, Philip and I played farming in the playground, pretty much in a world of our own.

At the first parents evening my teacher, Mrs Kinkler, asked my parents, *"Can Alan actually speak? Does he talk at home?"*

"Yes, of course he can," mum replied.

"Well, he doesn't speak in class, at all. He hasn't said a word all year!"

I struggled massively with learning to read, write, and spell, these days if I were in the school environment, I would probably have been told I had dyslexia. Mum, on the other hand, found all that easy and would often get frustrated with me, then one day something changed, and it was like she suddenly got me or understood me more. I found out years later that after she was sharing her frustrations about me to dad, he said, *"I know you find this stuff easy, but for me and Alan it's different. You read a sentence at a time, whereas we read a word or a letter at a time."*

Growing up on the farm it was not easy to meet and make friends due to the isolated location and my best friend at the time, Philip, lived on one of the farms on the other side of the road. Whilst it may sound close, it was still about two miles between our homes as the crow flies, or three by road. Either I was at his place or he was at mine. Though it felt a long way as a small boy, I was very thankful that we lived closer to each other than dad and his best friend from school, Allan, which took us ninety minutes to drive there to see him and his family. We went on special, annual, week-long family holidays with them, normally the first week of the summer holidays before the harvest started. There would be eight of us, my parents, myself and my sister, then Allan, his wife Ang and their children, James and Rachael, also a farming family. Year after year we went on holiday together, mostly to Bournemouth. Although we didn't get to meet each other often, we were all close friends and it was very inspiring to see that friends from school were still friends many years later. We also had a few weekends where we would meet up. When we were little, Rachel and I often talked about getting married when we were older.

It was not long after getting home from a trip after playing with Philip when I saw my dad crying in front of me for the first time. After a few minutes of feeling frozen with shock, I went to find mum and asked, *"What's wrong with dad? He's crying."*

"He's very sad because Grampy W unexpectedly died today."

Well, this was just as confusing for me, *"Ok umm, what does that mean?"* I enquired.

"It means he has gone up to heaven, as God wanted him up there. He is now at peace, the same as Grampy E a few years ago."

I didn't have many memories of Grampy E as I was only about two or three when he passed on. When I was a few years older, I also learned that Grampy died in dad's arms, they had been out to some agricultural meeting and his heart stopped with no warning.

I felt stupid not being able to make sense of what was going on and was scared of hearing more confusing stuff, so I didn't ask any more questions. A few weeks later, we had to go to a different church to our usual one, so we could bury Grampy's ashes. I had no clue what was going on after that, what were *his ashes?* Were they like ashes from the fire we had in the house during the winter? Why do we have his ashes if God had Grampy? All these questions were going through my head, but as most people were crying, I didn't ask, I didn't want to make them cry anymore. I didn't even say what I was told when I was crying; *"If you don't stop crying I'll give you something to cry about."*

The confusion didn't end there, about a year later, part of the farm and Gran's house was sold. After a few months of living in a small rented place, she moved into a bungalow in one of the nearby villages. Although I was mixed up; it was also like an adventure with a big garden and an orchard to explore. Later that year brought another adventure, with Mum taking myself and my sister away on holiday with my godmother, who was one of dad's cousins, and her three children, Paul, Andrew and Penny. This holiday was very different from all the others.

2

Get ME Out Of Here

Not only were we away with cousins instead of James & Rachel, but dad wasn't there, and we were staying in a caravan instead of a hotel – that all felt strange. We went to Plymouth on the south coast, home to the docks. I was a little nervous seeing all the big guns on the warships. Not far from the docks, was a little lighthouse except to a seven-year- old boy, it was massive, especially after we had climbed to the top circling round and round with every step. When it was time to go down, I was scared to death, I couldn't move, I cried and screamed in terror, and mum said something like, *"You're too big for me to carry you down, you'll have to walk."*

Not having another option didn't take the fear and panic away, I could only see a few steps and then nothing, scared that I might fall off after those steps. What mum didn't know was that just a few weeks before when I was playing at Philip's farm, I had fallen from a height. Philip and I wanted to join his two older brothers in a den they'd created on the top of a haystack. They climbed up using bale hooks, which are hand-held hooks that dig into the bales to give you something to grip onto. Struggling with the hooks, his brothers got us a ladder, but the ladder wasn't quite high enough. So, we climbed to the top of the ladder and they pulled us up to the top bale the rest of the way. Or at least that was the plan. Philip went first, but just before I got to the den, I lost my grip on the rope and landed in a heap on the floor. I didn't want to go to their den after that, although there was nothing broken, it was a very hard landing. My memory of how I got down is completely blank, even so, my mum has never let me forget that lighthouse experience and how I went up and found it almost impossible to get down.

Although the holiday was fun and enjoyable it didn't feel right without my dad. I missed him and was very pleased to get back to the farm and see him again. We were also back in time for the harvest, one of my favourite times of the year. I loved the smell of the fresh-cut straw as well as the opportunity to earn some pocket money by stacking straw bales on trailers. I first came across playing the guitar during this summer holiday, as somehow we ended up with Grampy E's old guitar at our house. I'm not sure if it had been hiding there for some time or if it was a recent arrival. We needed a musical instrument case for a comedy performance at Sunday School, where we had to take the instrument cases onto the stage, then inside each one, was a comb and a piece of greaseproof paper to make noise with. I felt this was daft and stupid and felt embarrassed to do it but as with many things I wasn't given a choice and was told I'd enjoy it when I got there. I never enjoyed Sunday school; it just felt wrong the whole time.

The guitar was an old classical one and I used to strum along not knowing anything about how to tune it let alone play it! The one song that I distinctly remember trying to play was *"The man's too big, the mans too strong,"* from Dire Straits, though I liked *"Money for Nothing,"* it sounded way too complex to just strum along to. After a couple of weeks of strumming an out of tune guitar, which probably sounded awful, not that I cared, we were over at Gran E's house and Auntie Marian, mums youngest sister, who played a classical guitar, was changing the strings on her guitar. I asked if I could have the old strings for Grampy's guitar and would she tune it for me? The following weekend Marian did this for me, then taught me how to play the G chord, although it was hard to get my fingers into position, I now knew something of playing the guitar and could strum along with Dire Straits with the one chord I knew on a tuned-up guitar. That made me feel cool, even though I had no clue what chords were being played on the song or that the guitar tuning would change from day to day and be affected by temperature. That period of me being a guitarist only lasted a few weeks, then it was back to the monotony of school.

Growing through the school primary years seemed to bring new changes every year, one difference was in PE - from running around inside the hall and jumping over things to going outside to play football in the winter and cricket in the summer. We did get a little bit of a head start as Philip's older brother Steven gave us a few lessons in their garden before going back to school. Even with this head start, I was never picked for the school teams, and for games in lessons and lunch breaks, I was always the one left until last, the one that was never good enough. This always made my heart sink and drained my energy. It felt like I didn't have any true friends even though I did have a few close friends. Philip had stopped going into assembly; when I enquired as to how he was getting out of it, he told me he had asked Miss Spicer, our teacher if she could teach him piano and that was the only time she could. That was it. I asked for piano lessons too, not so I could play, I didn't think it was as cool as guitar, but it got me out of assembly too.

Assembly, where the whole school congregated in the hall, often had songs, prayers and talks, normally from the headmaster Mr Owen, though he was fairly nice, he was a strict man. If someone started to interrupt his talks, he would lower his half-moon glasses on his nose, click his fingers and point at the guilty party, giving them a stern look, often this alone put the fear of God into a small child. We were not warned of what these talks were about or whether it would be Mr Owen or a guest speaker. Sometimes a fellow pupil would give a little talk if they had done something special, sometimes performing to demonstrate their musical abilities, such as playing the Star Wars theme tune on the piano or sharing a fund-raising activity. One week there was a guest speaker equipped with two big woven baskets with lids on that nearly came up to his waist. As I looked on with great curiosity as to what was in the baskets, simultaneously thinking that the contents would be very different from what could be found in Santa's Christmas sack. As he talked, he asked questions about fears that people may have and did anyone have a fear of the dark, noises, heights or spiders, and for each child to put their hands up if this were true for them. My hand shot up for heights and also the last one, snakes! Ever since seeing the James Bond film, Live and Let Die, where Bond is tied up and tormented by a witch doctor and a viper, I had been petrified of snakes, just like dad was. I couldn't even look at a picture of a snake in a book or on TV without being scared, feeling the hairs all over my body stand on end and my heart beating out of my chest. Just the mere mention of snakes and the idea that there could be some in his baskets scared the life out of me. He was saying how much of the time, a snake, spider or mouse would be more scared of humans than we are of them. Also that snakes don't eat or attack humans so there is nothing to be afraid of, which didn't help.

Then he took the lid off one of these baskets and pulled out a big snake! I just froze with fear I couldn't move, talk or anything. Some of the other children were volunteering to go to the front and touch them and allow them to coil around their necks. I so desperately wanted to run out of the room but I couldn't move. Some of them were asking questions about what they eat, or where they lived and if their skin was slimy, then one boy asked if the snake could crawl or slither around the floor. The speaker said that he didn't think the snake would move far on the polished floor surface but said he would put one down and see how it moved. That scared me even more, I believed it was going to come my way, luckily it didn't, just as the man said - it struggled to move.

At the end of his talk, the teachers got him to stand by the door of the hall, with a python around his neck and body and all the children were told to touch it as they went past. My sister and her friend went to speak to a teacher as her friend was scared of snakes too, they asked if her friend and I could go out the other door, but the request was refused. As I crept up to the door filled with terror, I could barely move and was pushed by whoever was behind me. I got to the door and stayed as far away from it as the door frame would allow. Its head seemed to come towards me with its forked tongue slithering in and out, reminding me so much of that Bond film - I ran from that door faster than I have run anywhere in my life.

I was teased by other classmates for the remainder of that year about my fear of snakes. I asked them to stop many times, though they never did; they just thought it was funny. I had nightmares about snakes for many years, both after the bond film and that school assembly. I only had a couple of years left in that school and just weeks of term before the holidays and being on the farm where I belonged. I was too scared to tell the teachers or my parents about the teasing I received, I just tried my best to ignore it and the kids doing it in the hope they would go away.

3

New Year, New Friends

The new school year separated Philip and I in class as he went up to the top class. They kept the less academic kids back in the same class and I felt like I wasn't good enough to go up with him. My sister and cousin Rachael had now gone to high school but my cousin Claire was still there in the top class in her final year.

There were two new boys in my class, Neil and Lee. I became good friends with both of them, it made a change for me to have friends who were not farmers. Outside of school, we would play a lot of football, which helped me to improve my skills as they took a little more time with me to help me learn and as I was not being pushed to the side-lines. They saw that I could play a little better than how I performed at school. Neil spoke to Mr Owen about this and I was then selected to join the school team as a reserve player a couple of times, but we lost both games and I wasn't picked again which made me feel sad.

Outside of school, mum also had me join the cub scouts, there were a few boys from school there of different ages. It helped me get to know some of the older boys as well as spending time with Lee, which did help my confidence a little. Spending time with Lee got me more into football and I started to support the same team that he did, Coventry City. They were one of the closest local teams and the company Lee's dad worked for were the team sponsors and he got to meet some of the players. One Saturday in 1987, when I was ten years old, we had to go on a cub scout trip to York, which was a long way from home. We visited the Jorvik Viking Centre (full of sickening smells) and the Railway museums which were both very interesting to young lads. This was also the day that Coventry City made it to the FA cup final for the first time in 104 years, so a doubly exciting day for us. Every shop window had TV's playing the City game and we were trying to catch up with what was going on.

That summer I had a challenge to complete, for my birthday I had been given a racing bicycle, it was not a new one; the paintwork was dull and rusty in places and it had no brakes and flat tyres with the rubber starting to lift off. Over the previous few months, I had rubbed the paintwork down, primed the paintwork and painted it red as well as putting new brakes on. After riding it for a while the tyres had almost disintegrated, especially after locking the back wheel up for a few skid slides, so they got replaced too. It may not have been a fancy brand, but to me, it had become a labour of love by giving me a sense of pride and achievement. It also gave me my first sense of freedom to run wild and run free. I may not have left the farm with it at that time, the main driveway alone was a mile long as was the rear-drive - that alone was enough space for a while.

Though I did fall off it; blaming the bike and saying I hated it for scraping my knees, ripping my jeans and on one occasion I ended up with a scratched face and torn lip. That was one of the two occasions I went home from playing on the farm feeling very sorry for myself with my tail between my legs. The other incident happened when my sister and I were playing with our cousins on the rock heaps halfway down the drive well out of sight of both sets of parents. I don't recall who came up with the idea of throwing stones, let alone why, but one of the stones my cousins threw hit me on the head rather nastily. I held my head where it hurt, then looked at my hand and found it had turned red. The stone had cut my head open and my hair was streaked red with blood, I screamed in pain and shock not knowing what to do and hardly able to move with my head throbbing. My sister rode her bike home as fast as she could to get our mum who came down in the car to pick me up. Once home, I was put in the bath to get cleaned up where the bathwater had turned red. Eventually, the bleeding stopped without a trip to hospital. We got a long talk on not throwing stones though. My cousins avoided that as we didn't want them to get in trouble, so it was kept quiet from their parents.

Of the four of us, myself, Christine, Rachael, and Claire, I was the only one who didn't take the 11 plus exam. Philip and I were the only two children in the whole school who did not get to take it. When our classmates would go off with Mr Owen for the extra tuition we would stay back in class and do other stuff. It gave me a feeling inside that I just wasn't clever and that the teachers and my parents didn't believe in me. Although Philip's older brothers were at the Grammar school and doing technical things that I didn't understand and didn't want to do, I still wanted to fit in with the other kids in our year. I just wanted to be like everyone else and to fit in.

My last year in primary school felt kind of strange being one of the biggest kids in school. I used to look up at the kids in the top class in their last year and think they were so grown-up yet there I was now one of them and didn't feel grown-up, let alone ready to go to the high school. Though there were two things I thought were positive about going to high school; one was that it was the last year in my life I would ever have to dance around the village maypole, which was so embarrassing, dancing around a pole with ribbons. The second was that it was another year closer to becoming the farmer I desired to be, as well as closer to the age of thirteen when the law said I was allowed to drive a tractor.

I had heard lots of stories from older kids about bullying at the high school; from name-calling to fist-fights and flushing heads down toilets. I was not looking forward to going there! Why could I not just walk away from school and work on the farm? I didn't need to get a school education, 'A' levels or a degree for that. During the Spring term, two of the teachers from the high school came out to speak to those of us who were likely to be going there, although for me it was a done deal whatever I said. As they talked, they mentioned the stories we had all been hearing and said that many of the stories were just stories about things that happened many years ago.

I was kind of torn over going to the high school, not just because of the bullying stories but also because Philip, who'd been pretty much by my side from nursery school was going to another school. I didn't like that idea, it felt like he was going to another country, not just another school.

4

Young Entrepreneur

In the summer holidays before starting at high school, I became an entrepreneur for the first time. Legally I needed to be thirteen to have a part-time job, so it wasn't an option for me. That aside, a paper round living where we did would have been a nightmare, as we were so cut off. I wondered what else I could do to get some extra pocket money.

One day at Philip's farm I helped him with some of his pocket money earners - collecting the eggs from the hens and cockerels and feeding them. After we fed them, he told me they were his to rear and sell, and that he got them from the chicken farm in between our farm and his farm. That night I asked dad if I could get some chickens to rear and sell also.

Over the next few days, we talked about where I was going to keep them and what and how I was going to feed them. I had all this worked out already, I'd keep them in one of the empty stables and screw some extra wood along the bottom of the door so they couldn't escape. I would feed them some grain that had overflowed from a truck being loaded with already sold grain that would only have gone to waste. I would make sure they were fed and watered before and after school.

To my surprise both parents agreed to it, as long as I did the work and sold them, I could keep the profits. Dad took me over to the chicken farm to see if I could buy some chicks. He also took me by surprise, *"Well, I think it's a good thing that young farmers get an early start, I have a few you can have, there's no charge, is it okay for me to drop them off to you tomorrow?"*

I looked at dad and he nodded at me, so I turned to the farmer and excitedly said, *"Yes please,"* though I also felt a little nervous as now I had to live up to my end of the deal. The next day he came over with fourteen chicks. I thought he would bring about five or six.

Over the next two months, I did keep up with it, although I hadn't expected them to be quite so noisy early in the mornings. I hadn't anticipated the door to the stable would be quite so heavy to open and close with the extra security on it. One by one, once they got to the right size, they were killed, plucked, dressed, and ready for the freezer. I had to get mum to help me with the dressing part as I didn't know how to do that bit, plus taking their insides out made me feel a little queasy. We kept two for our freezer and the rest I sold at £5 each to friends, mums, aunts, and uncles. Although profitable, I decided not to repeat it. I just thought there would be a better way for me even though I had no idea what it was.

Being at high school some things still didn't change, or if they did, they got worse. Even more than ever before, I felt like I didn't fit in. Like my world was condensing and getting smaller inside of me and out. Lee was the only boy from primary school that was in my class. There was only one boy who was a farmer's son in another class, so I didn't spend much time with him or have much of a chance to get to know him. This made me feel even more isolated and alone. In my class, there was another fairly quiet kid named Dan; he was a boy who had some kind of special needs or extra care and he was in a Special Needs group. I did go with him into that unit a couple of times during our lunch breaks. They were the only group in school that the school had computers for, and games to play. We did go to each other's houses a few times outside of school too. I felt comfortable in the CDT (Craft Design & Technology) lessons as it included woodwork, metalwork and practical things. Science and maths were OK, but I struggled with everything else. In fact, most of the time I was more interested in the tractor cutting the grass on the playing field than what the teacher was going on about.

I struggled with French; English words were hard enough to spell but to learn how to spell a word in French made it especially tough. The teacher was an old battle-axe who didn't understand why some pupils struggled with the language, and that probably didn't help me to learn. There was an opportunity to go to Erquy in France with the school, there was a big part of me that felt nervous and scared to go as I'd never been away from my parents for more than two or three days and this was a week and it would also be my first trip abroad. As Lee and Dan were going, I decided to go. During the trip, the teachers did some filming to make a video for the parents and kids to have as a memory or to see what their kids got up to. I spent most of the trip avoiding the camera, though I did get caught for about ten seconds twice. Mum did buy the video and probably thought it was a waste of money after seeing it!

Sharing a room with Dan, while away, was sometimes a little tense. He was obsessed with Arnold Schwarzenegger movies, most of which rated eighteen, even though we were only eleven or twelve. He quoted parts of the movies, especially the bits with swearing in and kicking and punching things which were over the top. He challenged Lee to a fist-fight in a classroom one lunch-time, which I didn't like. After that, I spent less and less time with Dan before he started to bully me. Most of the time it was lots of name-calling related to me being a farmer or living on a farm. He would say I was a *'sheep shagger'*, that I *'smelt of bullshit'* and that I lived too far away from anyone to have friends; other times he would kick chairs at me or kick me.

After a while, I did find the courage to tell our teacher and initially, nothing happened, then his Special Needs teacher got involved, as he'd had fights with other class members also. For a few days he calmed down, just the odd bit of name-calling, then his behaviour got worse again and he blamed me for him getting into trouble. One day he tried to push me down the stairs; just at that moment one of the older boys who went to the same primary school as I had, came around the corner and pinned Dan against the wall to stop him. He told Dan that if he bullied me again, then Dan would be bullied by him. It was a little confusing having someone else stick up for me, other than my older sister at times, as no-one else did. Dan didn't bother me much after that. Eventually, he spent more time in the Special Needs unit than in classes with the rest of us.

At the end of the first year in high school, I was caught completely by surprise by the news that Lee's dad's company had promoted him and moved his office from the Midlands down to South Wales. I wasn't looking forward to the next school year, as there would still be no Philip and now, no Lee. I couldn't help but wonder, would I have any friends the next year? It was pretty daunting feeling like everything important to me disappeared in some way, although I knew my sister would be there.

Having an older sister was sometimes very annoying, partly because she was older, partly because she was a sister instead of a brother; partly because at times she would introduce me to her friends as her, *"shitty little brother."* It was mostly the third shitty reason and I couldn't help but wonder what I had done wrong that made me seem such a shitty minor? A lot of the time I wasn't interested in anything she had to say but we both liked music of different kinds and different volumes and that was about the most common interest we came remotely close to. Over the summer holidays, our parents took us to Sidmouth, which for a teen is probably the most boring place in the world. Aside from nothing to do there of any interest - the beach doesn't even have sand! Why would you visit a sand-less beach? While there, I spotted someone wearing a t-shirt with what looked like an intriguing album cover on the front. I immediately needed to know more and asked my sister, *"See that t-shirt - who sings Guns n Roses?"*

She just said, *"You'll find out."*

The place we had lunch at later that day had a jukebox positioned in the corner of the lounge area that played music videos, which I didn't even know existed. It opened up a whole new world for me. Sis asked if she could put some music on.

"Just a couple songs," said mum.

She selected her choices, the first video pictured a band starting to set up for a concert, then she turned to me and said, *"This is Guns n Roses."*

I didn't get it but the lyrics referring to Paradise City, green grass and pretty girls stood out to me and I wondered if they too had been on holiday to Sidmouth.

One day during the summer holidays, sis burst into my room, *"You have to listen to this!!"*

"What is it?" I enquired.

"Iron Maiden," she said.

"I'm not into that heavy stuff," I said without knowing what they sounded like.

Ignoring my comment, she removed the cassette from my tape player, which was playing to the tune of Michael Jackson, pressed play on the new tape and walked out again. After I heard the first few chords played I kind of froze, there was something about it that wowed me and I couldn't switch it off, even though it was a little noisier than I was used to. I felt compelled to listen to the other side and was keen to see what album it was, but it was a copied tape and didn't say. I listened on, even more mesmerised. After it finished, I went into my sister's room and asked, *"What was that?"*

She just smiled at me, laughed, and said, *"Iron Maiden - the Number of the Beast!"*

I was hooked, just like that, and wanted more, much more. I didn't know what it was about the music but it was like I was transported to a different place when I listened to it, even more so than when I was younger and strumming along to Dire Straits. I didn't know much about them, just their music and the heavy reputation they had, for all I knew they could have just been on their first album and I'd heard all there was. To my delight, she said that they had released other albums, but she'd have to see if she could borrow some from her friends for me. One thing I was sure of, was that I had never connected to anything that quickly before.

A few days later she gave me another tape to listen to, and said, *"Here, this is Iron Maiden's first album, you may like and recognise Phantom of the Opera."*

"Opera? What? I thought they played guitars and rock music?"
"Just listen to it Alan!"

I didn't get this album as much as the other one, although two songs stood out to me from that first hearing, one being the *"Phantom of the Opera,"* which I recognised from a TV advert. To hear that played on a guitar, and at a speed I'd never heard before evoked something deep inside of me that I did not understand and that screamed out, *"I HAVE TO PLAY THIS ON GUITAR"*. The other song that I became fixated on was not so much because of the guitar music, but more because of the lyrics was, *"Running Free."* It was about a sixteen-year-old lad, who had no money or luck, I could instantly relate to that although I was nowhere near old enough to drive or to getting a pickup truck to run free and run wild. I felt magically connected to the tracks, it was like the singer had been where I was.

Throughout the rest of the holidays that year I listened to those two albums mostly, and some Guns n Roses, the more I listened to them, the more they grew on me, though still not on the same level as Iron Maiden. I asked my sister, *"Why do their guitars sound so different from that old guitar of Grampys we used to have?"*

"Because they're electric guitars."

I asked mum one day if I could get an electric guitar. *"Why do you want one of those?"* She enquired.

"Because I want to play Iron Maiden music on it," I said.

"Can you not just listen to it?" she asked.

"But I want to play the electric guitar, and I like this music," I said, trying not to show any disappointment. I didn't feel like I should ask again, or at least not the same day.

Although there was no electric guitar in my immediate future, it was my last summer holiday of not being old enough to drive the tractors. Although my thirteenth birthday still seemed so far away. I'd often wondered if I would be allowed to feed the cattle on that day or go for a drive in the fields or if I'd have to wait even longer. It would also be the first summer dad would be driving trucks instead of being on the farm.

We had trucks on the farm for a while by this point, initially cattle trucks, and then a grain truck all driven by my uncle. Dad preferred driving articulated trucks instead of the smaller rigid trucks. Dad went to drive for a small family firm that had a truck available, also being grain haulage and he enjoyed going out to other farms to load up. I loved joining him during the school holidays and at the weekend when the trucks would be maintained by one of the boss's sons. The four other trucks were driven by two of his sons, Chris and Mike, plus dad and another driver called Keith. At weekends I would help dad with cleaning his truck and help Chris with fixing them as much as I could. I found the workings of the truck fascinating and was quite surprised as to how I could just look at sections and figure out how it worked and asked Chris further questions to add to my growing knowledge.

Being in that environment led me to my next income stream, as the youngest I was naturally delegated as the one who needed to make the tea at weekends, so after a couple of weeks of getting to know people and putting the kettle on what felt like a thousand times, it became a pound a pot. It didn't matter to me who asked, I charged that fee to make a pot of tea or coffee and most weekends I came away with a tidy profit of £10 - £15. I daydreamed as to how many weekends would it take for me to have enough money to buy an electric guitar; my ulterior motive.

Once again, my sister came into my room, waving a tape in my face and insisting that I listened to it. *"What is it this time?"* I enquired.

"Metallica."

Although there was part of me that instinctively thought I was not into that heavy stuff, our other conversation popped into my mind and I decided I should listen to it before dismissing it this time!

5

Finally Thirteen

It was back to High school for the second year and back for more of the feeling of not having many options for where I would fit in. I didn't fit with the so-called *"cool lads"* as I didn't smoke or mess about in class. I didn't fit with the girls - although there were a couple I liked, I had no idea on how to talk to them; they might as well have been another species. I didn't feel like I fitted in with the geeks too much as I wasn't into computer games consoles, let alone trying to design my own game like they were during lunch breaks. One of the geek crowd I found also liked Iron Maiden; as did a couple of the lads in one of the other classes - one nicknamed Jon for being quite small, and one called Wiffy. Jon had a sister who was in the same year as my sister, so we had a few things in common. Wiffy was growing his hair and played the drums and was into many more bands than just Maiden. It stopped me from feeling quite as isolated.

I sat next to Jon in maths that year and we struck up a conversation. When he told me that he was having electric guitar lessons, I felt pangs of a little jealousy – that sounded awesome. During a visit to his house, he let me have a play on his guitar, I still remembered the one chord that I was taught years ago, and he showed me how to play another one. I was hooked. He showed me his sister's boyfriend's guitar that was there, an amazing red BC Rich Warlock in red. I'd never seen a guitar with such an unusual shape. I knew that I wanted one like that but in black, aware that it would be pretty expensive but just the thought of owning one and being able to play some of the music I was loving listening to, made my heart race!

I casually mentioned it to my mum when I got home, once again the response was less than supportive and not just from mum but dad and my sister also.

Mum said, *"But won't it be noisy and you don't know how to play?"*

Dad said, *"It could be a waste of money as your uncle had a guitar when he was young and someone sat on it and it broke."*

Sis said, *"It will be just like these other things that you played with a little and then didn't anymore."*

My heart sank and a feeling of disappointment set in, a little like Luke Skywalker in Star Wars when he wanted to go and be a fighter pilot, but his uncle said he had to stay on the farm year after year. A dream in the making dashed in one go.

Although I wanted to stay on the farm there was also a big part of me drawn to music. The big day arrived; I was thirteen years old and I could legally drive a tractor at last. I didn't get to drive that day as dad was out on the road driving the truck until late, though mum did let me go and start one and said, *"You have to wait until your dad's here to drive."*

I managed to get in a few short tractor drives, but it was pretty much on hold until the Summer school holidays. The time in between dragged on and on. With one week being very much like the rest, forced to go to school and hating it, going to the truck yard at the weekends and listening to music as much as possible in between half-hearted attempts at homework I had little interest in. I still completed the work as I thought if I started getting letters home from school I would be in trouble with my parents and having had a sore butt many times before, I didn't want another one. Not just because of the physical pain but also, and possibly more painfully, the feelings it produced of just not being good enough for them.

Most of my summer holiday was spent in the tractor cab, it felt like a dream being like my dad and after looking forward to it for so long. Even better - I was using it alone, and I drove up and down the field all day with an Iron Maiden tape blasting through the radio; I never wanted to go home. Most of what I did that summer was topping the Oil Seed Rape stubble to make it easier to plough, and power harrowing to get the ground flat so it was ready for the next year's crop to be planted. My first week was a little eventful, with having stones smash two of the windows, a puncture on the front of the tractor, and a puncture on the chopper. I thought I might have been told off for breaking things, but it was accepted as part and parcel of these things do happen. It was a bit blowy with the door window missing and was a good thing it was not during the winter months!

For some, driving backwards and forwards or round and round at slow speeds could be seen as boring - but not for me, I was coming alive as one of my greatest dreams that I'd lived out in my head was coming true. The rock star dream was still very much there, it just seemed like it had no chance of becoming a reality with no guitar to play. It didn't seem to matter as much when I was in the tractor in my own little world. In between singing or screaming along to my music I compared it to how much better it was than being stuck in a classroom and that I only had three years of school left before I would be on the farm full-time. The end was in sight!

6

All Change

We didn't see it coming and the big lifestyle change that was announced later that year caught me off guard and took the wind out of my sails. The farm was being put up for sale, four hundred acres of land along with our house. We were told that the farm wasn't making enough money to support us, my uncle and his family, and Gran.

If the farm had only been supporting one family household, not three, it would be different. Although I could understand the theory of why they were selling it. I had many questions whizzing through my head but I'd learned that sometimes I was better off not asking them, as I recollected the memory of my parents getting frustrated with me when I had so many questions about Grampy dying. Where will we live? Where are we moving to? Will we be moving schools too? What about my future of running our farm? What would dad do now? Would we have neighbours? What would it be like to have neighbours?

That farm was my future, the decision was made without anyone saying anything to me at all. More than anything else before. I felt that me as a person, my feelings, my dreams, and my future didn't matter to anyone. It was like my whole world had been squashed like an empty fizzy drink can with a big boot stomping on top of it - my soul had been crushed at that moment.

I didn't talk to anyone about it, let alone my opinion and feelings. I thought they should already know without me saying anything and talking would be futile. For my sister, it was more of an exciting possibility that we could move closer to some of her friends as she was more into going out with them than anything to do with the farm. I had grown up believing that farming was a way of life as opposed to making money but now it was being sold as it wasn't making enough. I couldn't comprehend how I felt or what these different sensations going on inside of me were, so I ignored them, pushed them down, and did what I was supposed to do - go to school and get an education.

It started to become more real when some of the potential buyers looked around the farm and our home. Before it was like a bad dream on the horizon, hoping I would wake soon and discover things were not so bad. The farm was sold in spring to the local water authority, who was interested in obtaining some of the fields to spread their recycled shit on when they couldn't sell it. The fact that they didn't even want to use it as a farm felt even more crushing. My uncle, who didn't want to farm anymore agreed to do the contract work and farm the land for a few years. They also wanted to rent out the house and as it needed some work doing to it before they could rent it through an agent, they agreed to rent it out to dad for six to twelve months.

In the early summer, it made sense why that one field only had half of it ploughed up and seeded for wheat. The half which was still grass was where the sale of all the farm machinery took place. I realised how long they had been talking about selling up before they told us, this just increased my feeling that I didn't matter. That feeling was so strong it prevented me from asking anything about the farm sale or anything related to it. In my mind, if I didn't matter, they wouldn't bother telling me anything else, after all, I was still just a kid to them.

Although I was still living in the same house on the same farm, it wasn't the same with the uncertainty of not knowing where we'd be living in a few months. I wasn't sure of my future path after I finally left school in a couple of years anymore. I just knew it was not to be a farmer as it would be wrong for me to work on someone else's farm.

I still enjoyed going to the truck yard at weekends and was learning lots there as well as gaining some good experience. I spoke to Chris a few times about becoming a truck mechanic after school, but I didn't want to go to college as I thought it would be like school that I hated so much. He persuaded me that college was different, and I could wear what I wanted and that much of what they taught was useful, unlike trigonometry, algebra and how to dissect a frog.

I felt a strong connection between where I was at in this period and to the lyrics of some Metallica tracks. Especially *"Dyers Eve,"* and *"Harvester of Sorrow"*, which led onto my forming a much stronger and deeper connection with music overall and increased my desire to play the guitar. I was passionate about reading about the bands I listened to in rock and the guitar magazines and watching live shows on video whenever I got the opportunity. I totally immersed myself in it all. Seeing the freedom of travelling on their tours, playing their music live and some of the shenanigans that some got up to excited my soul. To me, they were running wild and running free, I couldn't help but think and feel I would like to have a go at that.

Dave, one of my sisters' friends, had an electric guitar which he didn't play that often as he preferred to sing, so I asked if he would sell it to me but although he said no, he offered to lend it to me for a few weeks. I jumped at the chance, my class teacher played the guitar and offered me a few lessons during the lunch breaks. I jumped at that chance also.

Living on the farm without neighbours did have its benefits - I could learn to play guitar and not annoy the neighbours when I turned up the volume. It didn't stop my parents and sister complaining a little though. The other benefit was when it was party time- my sister had lots of them which had quite a reputation. Wiffy heard about them from dating a girl in my sister's year and said that next time we had a party to let him know and he would bring a live band along.

Usually, I went to stay at Gran's or friends to stay out my sister's way when she threw one of her famous parties - all of her friends would be drinking and I hadn't touched a drop of alcohol since the sherry incident. One of the last parties she had at the farm I did stay for, some of her friends coaxed me into sampling some beer and lager, which was okay but I was a little nervous that it may make me feel ill. My sister did try to stop me because if I hadn't had a drink, I was more useful to pick her up when she went out when we were older. Her intention backfired as it just encouraged me to try it even more.

I hosted one party there, it was a bit of a flop as I had heard rumours that a few others that I didn't like, trust or want at my house, were going to come and gate crash. I decided to tell some of the guests that it was cancelled, and made sure that only my close friends were told that it was still going ahead, hence only about ten people turned up, some of which were my sister's friends who were dating girls in my year.

That summer was the last time I got to work on the farm, which was in reality, just helping my uncle by doing some groundwork while he did the rest. With it being the first year of doing the farm on his own, it must have been hard, as it seemed like he was stressed or angry much of the time. Just the tiniest thing I did wrong or different to how he wanted, I was either yelled at or on the receiving end of a very abrupt message displaying his disgust and remarks on how I should have done it differently. Although I didn't like the way I was spoken to, I didn't say anything as I understood it was a stressful time of year, as well as remembering being told I needed to respect my elders when I was growing up. The tractor I was driving was an old Massey which he had hired in just for those six weeks, it had no radio, therefore no music, which made it feel very different to the year before.

Not long after that summer, we moved to one of the nearby villages, to a semi-detached country cottage, off a little lane. At the end of the lane was where my scout leader Colin, his wife Nina and their son Brett lived, although I had stopped going to cubs and scouts by this time. The house next door to us was occupied by a guy who was one of the top fuel dragster drivers, as he travelled all over the world racing, we only caught rare glimpses of him. One of the top drag race strips was close by, which was good because when they had the weekend races on they would often also have live rock bands play there as well as at the Bulldog Bash bike rally, and being locals, we were given free tickets to that. The Bulldog often had bigger bands playing for the Hell's Angels. The family who moved in after the drag racer moved out, Malcolm, Lisa and their two children Elli and George were much more sociable. It was an interesting experience living in a village and having neighbours quite a novel thing for us!

I was now on a different bus to school, so I didn't see any of the bullies that I did before and I continued to avoid them during school time. The journey each way consisted of trying to do some homework so I didn't waste home time doing it or listening to music on my Walkman while envisioning in my head that I was either at a Maiden concert or on stage with them. Exciting!

At home I'd either be listening to music in my room or trying to play it on the guitar I still had on loan from Dave, until there was a gig coming up he wanted to go to but he was short of money and decided to sell his guitar and amp to me to fund it. I had bought some guitar tablature books to go with it, which show you where to put your finger on which string if you can't read music to know which notes to play. I was in my element. My school teacher told me to get some books which showed chords and scales but I found them boring. I wanted to play the rock stuff, so I bought Iron Maiden's No Prayer for the Dying and Guns n Roses' Appetite for destruction. Though I couldn't play any of it as fast as it was played on the tape.

In my mind I felt like Dave Murray or Adrian Smith who were Iron Maiden's guitarists living the rock star dream but then when someone requested me to play something, I would freeze and everything I had learned seemed to disappear out of my mind at full speed, my heart rate paced rapidly, and I'd sweat and mumble – it was so embarrassing for how passionate I was about playing. Paul, I knew from school, had recently got himself a new guitar, which I tried out. He purchased it from Musical Exchanges in Birmingham, the new music teacher's husband's best friend worked there and gave him a good deal, and he encouraged me to speak to Mrs Atkins to see if I could do the same. I was scared to get rejected by her, but I very fearfully went up to speak to Mrs Atkins. I was also nervous as I didn't like new people. I saw Paul standing behind her nodding his head as if to say *"Do it, do it."* She was helpful and said that I needed to speak to Gaz, who was quite short, didn't have much hair and I'd notice that he has funny eyes. The curiosity of these funny eyes had me wanting to go to the shop almost as much as the pull of seeing lots of new guitars.

Jon's, and my parents agreed to us going. I think we may have forgotten to mention we were going to Birmingham city centre on the train. When Saturday came around, after a week that dragged, I met up with Jon, we walked around town for about twenty minutes before going to the train station to head off to Birmingham. I did feel a little nervous as it was the first time I'd been to a city without mum. It was reassuring as Jon had been there before with other friends and it was also exciting to have an adventure, as well as knowing there was a possibility, I could get a new guitar. I knew what I wanted, either a black BC Rich Warlock or a Jackson in dark red like the one Dave Murray had in one of the posters on my bedroom wall.

I felt a little more nervous on arrival as I was in a place I'd not been; my parents didn't know where I was and if I got a guitar, how would I explain it to my parents? I'd not thought about that bit! Then there was having to walk into a shop and ask to speak to this Gaz guy, instead of my normal walk in, look around, and if someone comes to me say *"oh, it's okay I'm just looking,"* and escape. After a ten-minute walk we were there and peering into the shop it looked massive and thrilling. As soon as I was through the door, I felt like my eyes popped out of their sockets, the only music shop in Stratford had a guitar section with about 4 classical guitars and one acoustic but no electrics. Here, the back wall was covered in guitars, three or four high, and continued as far as my eyes could see. Had I died and gone to guitar heaven I wondered for a moment?

After a couple of minutes of standing there, in a trance-like state, a long-haired guy came up to us. Jon stated that he could help me, pointing towards me. Still slightly mesmerized by all the guitars I mumbled, *"Umm err Gaz, I'm looking for Gaz."*

He said, *"Well, I'm not Gaz, I'm Steve. Give me a minute I will get him for you."*

As I gazed around, the only person in the shop with short hair was me, which made me question if Gaz was around. When Steve walked back up to us, he stepped to the side and behind him stood a short man with little to no hair and funny looking eyes, they kind of looked like they could pop out of his head at any moment - I couldn't help but think it could be as a result of working around all these guitars. Gaz introduced himself, so I told him why I was there. He said to browse and find the guitars I'd like to try and Steve would get me set up in the soundproof room. When

I found the axe that I felt fitted me the best, he'd sort me a deal out. We walked around, my heart was still racing, not knowing which way to look as I was spoilt for choice. Then, in the corner of my eye, I spotted a blue BC Rich Firebird, and as I got closer to it, just behind it was a Warlock and it was black!

My initial thought was, *"Wow, that is going to be mine,"* then I saw the price and my excitement waned as it was nowhere near my price range. Regardless, I asked Steve if I could have a go on it and got set up in the soundproof room. It felt great to play, even better than I remembered. I enquired about Jackson as this one was a bit more than I could afford. Steve explained that Jackson's are a similar price to this, but they had a Japanese Warlock which was cheaper than the American model I had in my hands; a grand cheaper. I asked if I could play the Japanese one as it was very similar and played just like the other one. I played it for nearly an hour and fell in love! Steve came back and said that I took longer to choose than anyone else. Gaz knocked about £40 off it for me and gave me a hard case for half price; it was a dream come true. I was now the proud owner of a black BC Rich. Grinning from ear to ear, I knew this would help me to sound and play better but then my thoughts flipped back to how I was going to explain my new guitar to my parents.

7

Tears in Heaven

Back at home with my guitar, I thought I may get told off for wasting my money but to my surprise mum was interested in why I hadn't mentioned the trip to Birmingham. It shouldn't have surprised me as she hadn't been impressed by the time I went to Stratford on my bike from the farm and told her afterwards. She asked why on that occasion too, well, it was because she would stop me from going, so I just did it anyway as it meant so much to me.

I did feel a little bit cooler with my new guitar, even if I still didn't know how to play but learnt quite a bit from jamming with my friends at lunch-time and occasionally at each other's houses. One of the six formers on the school bus came to my house to jam a couple of times until he started dating my sister. I did wonder if he just used jamming sessions with me to come to the house and get to know her better. One night during half-term they had gone out together and then called the house late, at about eleven-thirty. It did seem weird, them phoning when they had gone out, especially at that time and asking to speak to me. I suspected it was some kind of wind up as I walked to the phone in my parent's bedroom.

As soon as I heard my sister's voice I could tell it wasn't a joke, it sounded serious from her tone, *"Your friend from school, the one who plays the drums - Wiffy is dead."*

I just replied with a rather numbing *"Ok, thanks for telling me."*

He was fifteen years old; how could he be dead? What happened? I didn't know how to feel. I just had too many questions with no answers, my mind was in turmoil. I climbed back into bed, not feeling real. I knew my parents wouldn't have any answers either, so I didn't ask. Mum came to my room, I think she felt it was weird my sister calling me that late, to see if I was okay.

"Wiffy's dead," I said.

She said she was sorry to hear that and asked if there was anything she could do?

I knew she couldn't bring him back, so I just said no and pulled my duvet cover up over my head and as I heard the door shut, I started to cry. So much for, *"Big boys don't cry."* I thought to myself, *"Why am I crying when I keep hearing people say big boys and men don't cry?"* I had no idea what was going on inside of me or how to explain it to anyone even if I wanted to talk about it. I wouldn't know where to start. And how would talking help anyway? I wondered if there was something wrong with me. Maybe I wasn't good enough to be a man? So many questions to which there were zero answers, leaving me all the more utterly baffled and a sense of unworthiness, although I couldn't put my finger on that either exactly. It was all vague yet very uncomfortable.

Wiffy and I were the only lads in our year who had grown our hair and without him I was going to feel like the odd one out, but Iron Maiden, Metallica and all the bands I was into had long-hair so I didn't want to get it cut. Even the comments about being a girl because of my hair hadn't put me off previously.

Back at school the following Monday, there were a few other sad faces in class and an assembly was arranged for our whole year group. The deputy head addressed us all and informed us all about Wiffy in case anyone didn't know about his death. Then he said there had been many rumours going around that he may have taken his own life and that this wasn't the case. From what the parents had told the school, he was on some antidepressant drugs which were believed to have been too strong for him and his heart had stopped. I hadn't heard the suicide rumour and wouldn't have believed it if I had, he always seemed happy whenever I saw him and was doing well with his drumming, having been a part of a couple of bands as well as the school theatre show, which was about to go on a small tour with the RSC. Another teacher read a poem that Wiffy had written, then two other teachers played their acoustic guitars and sang the Eric Clapton song, Tears in Heaven and dedicated it to Wiffy, both trying not to cry as they performed.

The funeral was to be held in the biggest church in town, it was on a school day but students in our year were allowed to wear a black tie that day and attend the service if they had a letter from their parents with their permission. Anytime I had asked if I could be out of school for any reason in the past my parents had said no, so I figured this would not be an option, so I didn't bother asking.

My class teacher said that the school band that Wiffy played drums in were going to do a couple of gigs at other schools to raise money to help contribute towards a tribute for Wiffy. His older brother was going to play drums for them and our class was asked if anyone else would like to contribute in some way. I volunteered but had no clue what I could do, although I wanted to be in the band, I couldn't actually play any single songs, let alone a whole set-list. We did three gigs between two schools; the first went down so well they invited us back for another gig. I helped mainly with setting the gear up at the beginning of the evening and stripping down after the show, with my first introduction to sound engineering in between.

The band consisted of two teachers playing guitar and pupils playing bass and on vocals, with Wiffy's brother on the drums. It did seem a little strange seeing someone else in Wiffy's place. It was the first time I had been to a rock concert and I loved the environment with the loud guitar music and being able to be part of it made it extra special and increased my desire to see Iron Maiden live. It fuelled my dreams of one day being able to play in a live band myself.

At the first show, during the second half, a slim, pretty, long-haired girl came up to me and asked me if I wanted to dance. Me dance? I didn't know how to dance and every time I had tried, I just felt stupid and the memories of being forced to dance around the maypole in primary school flooded back. I turned her down and she went away with her friends again. I was so scared of embarrassing myself or tripping me or her over, let alone having people laugh at my dancing. After the show, the sixth form girl who did most of the singing looked at me and called me a heartbreaker, then asked if I had any idea how hard it was for a girl to walk up and ask a boy to dance. She then asked if I found it easy. Umm no, that's why I had never done it. Apparently, for a girl it was even worse, she was possibly thinking she was not pretty enough. That made me feel sad, it was like my heart dropped from my chest to my toes. I hadn't stopped to consider that in my total fear of embarrassment.

At the second show, there was a blonde girl in the crowd and I heard via her friends that she fancied me. I did not believe it at all, I couldn't see why a girl would fancy me without getting to know me. I was just a teen with acne all over my body and long hair that no-one seemed to like and looked nothing like any of the celebrity heartthrobs that I heard the girls at school raving on about all the time. I assumed it must have been some kind of joke or wind up but why would they do that? Girls were just so confusing to me, almost as if they were from another planet. As far as I could tell, none of the girls at school fancied me, or if they did, they were trying to tell me with telepathy or something and I just wasn't getting the message.

It wasn't just girls that I was struggling within school, as it got closer to taking my GCSE's I found nearly all of the lessons a struggle - not being able to do my work as fast as the others and not understanding what the teacher was on about half of the time. I didn't care as I had already decided which lessons I was going to put some effort into; Science as I could achieve two qualifications for one subject, Maths, because I found numbers easier to understand than words and CDT (Craft Design and Technology) as it included woodwork & metalwork and was practical and involved far less writing. They were also the subjects I needed to pass to get into college and study truck mechanics.

In CDT I had to make three things in the two years of study, one project was a wall clock so I created a Metallica clock; the next was something to do with Leisure, so I made a guitar stand and the third project had to be connected with lighting. Sometimes the CDT would let us play music when we were doing the practical. I got to choose some music to play one week, it just happened to be the time Iron Maiden released their latest album, *"Fear of the Dark,"* and as with all of Maiden's music, I loved it. As part of the promotion for the album, they were doing one show in England that year by headlining the Monsters of Rock festival at Donington Park. I wanted to go but last time they played there, back in 1988 with a crowd of over 100,000 people and sadly two people died.

I thought long and hard about asking my parents if I was allowed to go; it wasn't just that they might not let me go because of what happened in '88 but also getting there and back safely and the cost of the ticket. I thought they may say no. One day I spoke to Brett, our neighbour's son, knowing he was also a Maiden fan and went to a lot of gigs and being a few years older with a driving licence. I asked him if he was going to Donington and if he was, could I possibly get a lift? He said he wasn't sure and would let me know. After that, I thought it may be best to say something to mum in case he did, and I briefly mentioned it.

A few weeks later he confirmed that he would be going and would give me a lift if I still wanted to go, as long as my parents were happy. Much to my surprise, when I asked, they said yes! What I didn't know at the time was that Brett had spoken to Nina, who said he had to ask my mum if she was happy for me to go with him, before he told me that I could. I found it hard to believe that in three months, not only was I going to a real gig but it was Maiden that was headlining along with another five bands playing and I liked all of them. It felt like it would be a very long time between now and the actual day. The time flew, between being with my music in my bedroom, with dad at the truck yard or stuck at school.

For two weeks I did get to be out of school for work experience, which took place at the local tractor garage. One of the biggest lessons was the absolute certainty that I didn't want to work there when I left school. The work and the job itself were okay, I also learned that I was more interested in fixing trucks than tractors. However, there were a couple of guys working there that my personality clashed with theirs. One of them just didn't get me having or wanting my hair long, let alone my interest in rock music.

In a way, I was pleased to be out of there and back to school; that was a first! I got introduced to another Iron Maiden fan in school; he was in the year above me and his hair was about three times longer than mine, he was into his art and also doing CDT with rock and metal music inspired projects. He was also going to Donington to see Maiden. I did wonder if

I would see him when we were there, though from the crowded pictures of previous shows I thought it would be unlikely.

The summer holidays finally came around, but it was still five weeks until Donington. Our family holiday this year was going to be a little different. Not only were we going away with Allan, Ang, James and Rachel for the first time in a few years, but we were also going abroad for the first time, to Tenerife. I had not been on a plane before and was feeling a little apprehensive about it after all, I was scared of heights and planes went up way higher than I had ever been before.

Despite those few nerves, I was looking forward to going on holiday with James and Rachel again. I had my Walkman and tapes with me as well as I didn't want to go a whole week without my music and leaving behind my guitar was bad enough. Luckily, I found that flying for me was okay as I couldn't see the drop below, although the plane shaking about with the turbulence did make me hold on to the seat a little tighter than I was before. After it happened a few times I thought it must have been normal as the hostess' just carried on handing food and drinks out in a very calm way, not to mention the plane didn't fall out of the sky. That was a big relief as any plane crash on the TV or movies looked pretty scary.

We took two taxis from the airport and after two and a half hours of going around a one-way system we were all wondering why they hadn't dropped us off yet, I just wanted to go to sleep. I'd had enough by then and dad claimed that we were never going abroad again. Then our driver finally had the sense to ask at one of the other hotels where our resort was. It turned out we had given him the new English name for the resort which had just opened and previously they were holiday apartments with a Spanish name. Once he had that, we were there within five minutes.

8

Can We Get Off The Bus?

The Resort manager had stayed an extra two hours to welcome us after he should have finished as the reception had closed. After a few hours of sleep, we got up to go and explore, after arriving in the middle of the night. It was amazingly warm, I'd never felt heat like it, yet there was a nice cool breeze that came from the sea over the golf course.

The first couple of days consisted of our parents lying in the sun while we would swim, play games and indulge in a little sunbathing. Lunchtimes were extended so dad and Allan could have a few beers, followed by more in the evenings. The couple that ran the pool bar, Louis, and Maria, treated us like friends, they couldn't do enough for us. Even when Allan joked about it being happy hour, Louis would agree and dropped the prices for a while. On day three we hired a minibus to take a trip up Mount Teide; Allan was driving it even though the steering wheel was on the wrong side and we had to drive on the wrong side of the road, it didn't slow him down, neither did being partially blind in one eye! Jeez…

The direction that we must have taken was the most scenic and off the beaten track route on the island. At one point we turned around and once back on the right road we could see the track we were on and if we had kept going we would have come to a sudden stop as there was a bridge over a stream that had collapsed. Even the road we were on wasn't great with being very windy and not having any visibility as to what may be around the bend. Sitting on the passenger side of the bus, mum and I could see a clear and very real view of the sheer drop down each side of the mountain as if we were about to fall off. Hair raising didn't come close to it.

We finally reached the top and whilst walking around, it looked like being in one of the Star Wars film locations. Seeing the patterns in the rocks caused by the volcano eruptions I was fascinated and could have stared at them for hours as they were a natural beauty, I had not seen anywhere else before. Or was it just a relief to not be on the bus, unsure of whether we may fall off the roadside? It was a wild journey. On the way back down, the other side of the road was more like a proper road which felt a lot safer. It did seem kind of bizarre how the side of the island we were staying at was like a desert, yet the other side was like a rainforest.

There were a lot of other families staying at our resort and one day Ang asked if I had seen the talent. I had to ask what she meant, I wasn't sure if she was referring to Nigel Benn the boxer, known as the dark destroyer, who was there with his lady and little child, whilst he was training for an upcoming fight. She explained that she was referring to whether I had seen two pretty girls that were there. I noticed them the first day but as with many pretty girls, they caught my eye, but I had no idea what to do with them or how to talk to them. They were the other species. I acknowledged that I had noticed them but didn't continue with the conversation as I didn't want to show how useless I felt around girls I liked, all while I cringed inwardly.

During the week, James started talking to one of them, I followed and talked a little with the other girl, believing there was no way she would be interested in someone like me as she was far too pretty and could be with any boy she wanted. Even though they were both friendly towards both of us, I didn't see much point in trying to be anything more. They had told us to start with that they were from Germany, though it eventually turned out that they were from Cardiff and just faking foreign accents. I couldn't help but wonder if they were lying about where they came from, what else were they lying about? It didn't feel very respectful, maybe we should have noticed their suspect accents earlier? After finding out about the lies, I spent more time plugged into my music, especially the music from the bands that were playing at Donington the following month. I wanted to make sure I knew all of the lyrics to all of their songs ready to sing along. Music was a great way for me to not only escape from the world around me but also to feel different. When I was plugged in, not having a girlfriend, or believing I could get one, plus the feelings of not being good enough, dissipated and it was like nothing else mattered or even existed to a degree.

On the last night, Louis and Maria offered to cook a paella for us all but the idea of what was in it just made me feel sick without even eating it; my sister wasn't overly impressed at the thought of it either. The frying pan Louis used to cook the paella was as big as one of the tables in the bar. It was just for our two families and everyone else just watched. He rustled up a steak for me and my sister which was the best steak I had ever tasted.

I liked Tenerife and didn't want to leave it behind, especially the weather. The tan I gained hid the acne that I had all over my chest and back. no-one was bullying me or picking on me so I could relax there. I hadn't been anywhere like it before, though I did miss not being able to play guitar. I had my imagination though, as I listened to my Walkman, my fingers were moving as if I had a guitar in my hands. I was sure some people looked at me and thought I was a freak in some way. I know I thought that when I looked at myself in the mirror.

No-one else wanted to leave the next day either, even dad, who said we were never going abroad again loved it and didn't want to go home. The taxi trip was a lot faster this time. I wondered why holidays had to only be a week; why couldn't they be two weeks, a month, or a year?

Arriving home felt kind of sad. I was excited about the Monsters of Rock festival but that was still four weeks away. I wasn't working on the farm this year and didn't quite know what to do with myself over the school holidays. I played guitar and listened to music a lot and I did go out in the truck with dad a few days, even then, some of the time while he was driving, I was still plugged in. Those four weeks went faster than I could have ever imagined.

9

Running Free

The Big day finally arrived, not only was it my first time going to the Monsters of Rock, some of the band members were going for the first time too. I heard the guys in Skid Row saying in a radio interview on the rock show that they used to look at the album sleeve for Rainbow's Live at Donington, which displayed a picture of the crowd taken from stage and dream about what it would be like to play there. That sounded familiar to me as that was the same thing I did with the Iron Maiden pictures.

We left nice and early in the morning, although I hated early mornings today, I didn't mind one bit! Brett brought one of his Uni friends along so the three of us travelled with rock music blaring out the stereo, they were talking about Uni stuff in the front, so I just listened to the music, disappearing into my own little world and letting them get on with it. When we parked the car and walked to the arena, we agreed on a place to meet between the bands if we got separated in the crowds, there were no mobile phones in those days so it was the only way.

The crowd was made up of all sorts of people, not just in looks but also ages, the eldest was around seventy and some couples had even brought their kids along, which surprised me as my parents wouldn't be seen dead there, let alone alive. The first band of the day came on, The Almighty, we were about halfway to the front of the crowd and heard the first few bangs of the drums on the first track, even before the guitars came to life and the whole site just seemed like it had been electrified and thousands of rock fans came to life at once. I had never experienced an atmosphere like it and I loved it, I wanted more. I couldn't help but wonder if it felt this good with the Almighty what would Maiden be like? There was a bit of The Almighty's set which didn't quite make sense at the time, the singer wanted to introduce a *"new man"* and started going on about Wayne's World and Canadian Club Whisky. I wondered if he used to be a woman and had a sex change after too much to drink, either way, I didn't care, I liked their music and decided to buy some of their tapes.

All the bands playing were enthralling, although there was part of me that would have loved it even more if Metallica were there instead of Slayer. My favourite bands of the day were Iron Maiden, Skid Row and the Almighty. It felt like everyone was there for the same reason, to have fun and enjoy the music as if everyone was one big happy rock family. no-one was trying to be better than anyone, no bullying and none of the guys was getting the *"You look like a girl with your long hair,"* comments. Everyone seemed to understand and respect each other.

The atmosphere when Iron Maiden came on went into overdrive, as it was better than I had even imagined, my excited senses went wild! When they came on stage blasting out *"Be Quick or Be Dead,"* there was a massive surge to the front from pretty much the whole crowd. The three of us had stayed fairly close together up to that point but after that, I couldn't see either of them. It didn't worry me too much as I knew we had agreed to meet afterwards back at the car. A few favourite songs I was hoping that they would play were; Phantom of the Opera, Hallowed be thy name, Running free, Wasted years, Mother Russia, Wrathchild, Aces High, and the Trooper. They played four out of that list, though the one moment that stuck in my mind was when they played Running Free, as they had Adrian Smith come on stage to play the song with them, he left the band two albums before. I had never seen or heard of a band playing with three guitar players before, it was completely unexpected which made it all the more exciting!

Other than the mad surge at the start of the Maiden set, I hadn't considered how many people eighty-two thousand was or how much of a challenge it would be to get myself out of a crowd that size. Even after the music had stopped, the noise from the crowd screaming for more was intense, so asking someone to please move, was a little tougher than I expected. Would I get out of there before sunrise, as it was 11pm. now, I wondered? I found that although going across to the side was the shortest route, going backwards was the easiest method, as the further back I got, the fewer people I had to push through. My heart was racing like crazy;

I don't know if that was down to the adrenaline rush of the show or the fear I may not get home.

I found my way back to the car park, stumbling in the dark through a field with little light was a little tricky. Had I gone the right way and was I in the right field? I pondered as I walked round and round and up and down, although mobile phones did exist, they were like a suitcase with a receiver and no-one would have taken one of those to a rock concert. After feeling like I had covered the whole field and not found the car once again, I started to panic a little as I wondered if I would ever get home that night. They wouldn't have gone without me, would they? I doubted that they would do that. Then at the back of the field, I discovered there was a gate through to another smaller field with a lot fewer cars parked up. I figured I had nothing to lose by checking them out too and the first car I came too just happened to be the one I had been looking for, bingo, for what seemed like a two-hour search. They were both waiting for me, which was a bit of a relief, but then we queued for another hour or so to get out of the car park and onto the road to get home. We relived the evening as we queued, Bret asked if my ears were ringing? They were and he explained it was the effect of loud music and it would stop by the following day but that's why when you go to gigs, especially indoor gigs, you need to wear earplugs and it would be a good idea not to use your headphones for a day or two to let your eardrums recover.

By ten o'clock the following morning, my ears had stopped ringing just as Bret said they would. I didn't use my headphones either but continued to play music loudly in my bedroom. After a few days the buzz within me from seeing the bands I had imagined watching live for a couple of years, had dropped off a bit and the reality of going back to school in just over a week hit. It was a draining thought even though it was the school year I had been looking forward to for many years, the last one ever.

This term I had a few different tales to tell from previous years, not that I was expecting anyone to ask, as in school I pretty much kept myself to myself and didn't let anyone in. No-one understood me or liked me. I assumed most people just thought I was weird or boring as I wasn't into any of the things they were, I believed that of myself too, so I didn't try to fit in other than with my few friends that also had a hint of weirdness.

The third and final CDT project was about to start, having made a Metallica clock, and a guitar stand for the leisure project, now I had to create something with lighting. I had the options of using wood, metal and plastic, and had looked into a light show for a rock concert but it would have been a little challenging to have examined and prove that I had created it. I went to the lighting shop in town to see if I could get some inspiration or new ideas. They had already had several pupils through the doors, and they said pretty much all they could suggest, was to make a desk lamp.

I felt the same about that project as I did about fitting in with anyone in school, it didn't feel right to me. I told the teacher I wanted to make an electric guitar, she laughed for a few minutes before realising I wasn't joking. She thought I was completely and utterly bonkers, but she knew I meant it and said, *"Your brief is to make something to do with lighting. If you can find a way to do that and stick to the process with designs and plans that you need for the exam board, I can't stop you, just make sure no-one gets electrocuted."*

That was all the permission I needed, I had something in mind and a plan to implement. I dug out my old second-hand guitar that hadn't been used since I got my BC Rich, and used the neck and electrics from that, then took a trip to musical exchanges to get some advice on where and how to mount some of the pieces onto the body and get it set up. I did ask my parents if I could go this time though. There was an old door in the CDT room which wasn't going to be used again so I cut it in half and glued it together to form the body. I wanted a shape that was halfway between a Gibson Explorer and a Flying V but with curves.

By the time I had done all this, my classmates thought I was bonkers too, *"What the hell has that got to do with lighting?"*

I heard it many times. When the body was finished it was painted black and within the front surface of the body were three strips of LED lights, all flashing in sequence, controlled by a circuit board I had created with a little help from my class teacher who was also the head of physics. Outside of school, I got asked about it also as Philip's older brother had called to see if I wanted to join the Young Farmers club that he was chairman of at the time, and they were having a new members evening. I went along with him and Philip, which I did enjoy as it seemed I fitted in a little more than at school, though at the same time, I felt like I didn't fit in as we no longer had our farm. A couple of the other members my age were also taking CDT and were making desk lamps.

Towards the end of the year, during the exam revision period, there were a couple of days each week we were allowed to go into school to finish uncompleted projects. For me, this was my guitar project. It was a little strange working in the workshop with limited supervision with a class of first or second years, under the watchful eye of the teacher. Luckily, I got it finished in time, with it all working as intended, including the essential lights. The only real issue being that when the flashing lights were switched on, the pick-ups on the guitar would also pick up on the microchip that controlled the lights as well as the notes played.

Joining Young Farmers was good for me as it got me out of the house and meeting people, including a few that were into the same music as me which did make things a little easier. I organised for five of us to see Iron Maiden in Birmingham together. Although it was two of the bands from Donington (Maiden and the Almighty) it was an indoor gig and was a very different experience. For a start, it seemed much louder with the sound bouncing off of all of the walls and ceiling. I felt the beat of every bass drum kick and some of the bass guitar pulsing through my body. We were seated as the standing tickets were all sold out, all the band members looked pretty small from where we were so I watched the big screens a lot and hoped they would show what the guitarists were doing with their hands more than the singers face.

Ricky, the singer of the Almighty, announced they had just been added to the Metallica gig at Milton Keynes Bowl in the summer, I had already had my tickets ordered. I was looking forward to seeing Metallica as well, and now the Almighty and Megadeth were also to be on the same stage for the first time since Metallica had kicked out Dave Mustaine, who then formed Megadeth, with a lot of bitterness between the two bands. I didn't think the two bands would ever play at the same festival, let alone on the same day, one after the other.

For my first few months in Young Farmers, I refused to go to any of the disco's that were put on by various clubs around the county. The first one I ventured to was our own, as I was encouraged to support our own club. I wasn't looking forward to it as I didn't dance. I was not into disco music at all and didn't believe that any of the girls would be interested in me either, so what was the point?

The disco wasn't as I expected as most of the night the lads were standing by the bar chatting and drinking, the girls would drink a little before hitting the dance-floor, and none of them asked any of the lads to dance. I noticed that once some of the lads had a few drinks they did venture onto the dance floor towards the end of the night and I wasn't the only one who had no idea how to dance but the feeling that I should not be on a dance floor, even after a few drinks, wouldn't shake off. I enjoyed it enough to go to a few more.

10

Finally Out Of School

During my free periods, I chose to partake in some interviews and skills tests. I had a reserve place at a car college too for a full-time mechanics course but I wanted to be learning hands-on and not in a classroom. I'd had enough of that. One of the skills tests was with the Warwickshire Garage Training Association (GTA).

After my tests, the assessor asked me to stay behind, I thought she was going to tell me I had failed and everyone else had passed. But she asked me if I was dyslexic. I said, *"I don't know as I have never had any tests, I just thought I wasn't as smart as other kids as implied and suggested by many teachers."*

"Well, that is not the answer I was expecting, how do you think you did?" she replied.

"Umm, I'm not sure, probably not too well as I'm the only one you kept back," I said quietly, hoping the ground would just swallow me up and get me out of there.

"Well, the reason I asked about dyslexia is that you took longer to answer all the questions than the others. Some of the challenges you hadn't finished by the end of the allocated time but then everything you have answered was with 100% accuracy, so we will be putting you forward for apprenticeship interviews. What kind of garage would be your preference?"

I stood there for a minute or two just trying to take in what she had said, *"Umm, Trucks please,"* I said.

I didn't know what else to say, though I did wonder if prospective employers would look at my uncompleted test results the same way. Having already had one interview for a construction, design and engineering company and performed quite poorly in the interview, I was more than a little nervous for future options.

An offer of an interview came through with a local transport firm that used to come and collect the milk from our farm when we had the cows. When it came to the day, I didn't wear a suit as I never felt comfortable in them and for a job where I was just going to get dirty I thought it was silly. Mum gave me a lift there and waited in the car for me, I went in with my palms sweating, my heart racing and butterflies in my stomach and nervously asked for the man called Bob that was printed on the appointment letter I had in my shaking hand. After a few minutes of what felt like an eternity, Bob came in and introduced himself and said that he was just the contact person and I was going to be interviewed by the CEO. At that point, I wanted to scarper but I wasn't sure if my legs would work and I shuffled into the CEO's office behind Bob, the CEO was a much older man, in his seventies.

The CEO got his secretary to make us a cup of tea and he asked me what I knew about the company. I searched my head that felt pretty empty right then but remembered they started with collecting milk and had been trading for a long time. He filled me in with more about the company. He then struck the fear of God into me and said, *"I have been reading your report and information from the GTA and I have some questions."*

Yikes, I felt my whole body drop to my shoes thinking he was questioning if I would be good enough for the job.

"It says here," he started reading it out loud, *"you're a member of the Young Farmers club."*

He shared a little about his days in young farmers, *"I have to ask - you're a Watts and in Young Farmers, with the area you live, do you know of a Berty Watts?"*

That caught me off guard and grounded me a little, *"Yes I know the name, he was my grandfather but he died a long time ago."*

Although school had given us some basic interview tips I wasn't prepared for any of that.

"Well, my boy," he said, *"I remember Berty from Young Farmers and many other times after, he was a very good man. Tell me about your mum's side of the family?"*

I said that they still had their dairy farm, not far from their original yard.

He then stood up, walked over to pick up a phone on the side counter and called someone, *"Bob, we will be okay with this young man, I went to Young Farmers with his grandfather, we used to pick up milk from both sides of his family,"* He looked at me and asked, *"Oh you will be taking the job won't you?"*

Slightly shocked, I nodded, as I didn't think any words could come out of my mouth in those few moments.

He then personally escorted me out of the building as he wanted to meet my mother. Mum was quite surprised by that, he revealed that I had got the job and that he had high hopes for me. Mum said, *"Oh, he is very keen to learn."*

The CEO then said, *"I can tell he is, with how far he has come to get to this point, some kids just aren't interested."*

They also talked about farming and our families a little before he went back inside and arranged for me to be taken to their workshop, look round and meet my manager on another day.

Although I wasn't going to start until after we had our holiday, I was pleased and relieved that I had an apprenticeship and knew what I was going to be doing for the next three to four years even if I failed all my GCSE's. For me, school was done and all that remained was to return some books and say goodbye, or good riddance, to my teachers. Some of them asked me if I was going to stay on and do my A levels, I thought, *"Wow, you don't know me do you?"* I felt proud to say that I had an apprenticeship. They then told me that I needed to have A levels and a degree to be successful but went very quiet when I asked them why?

The next trip to Tenerife was also a bit of an adventure, even though we had a good idea what to expect, as it was the same resort as the year before. I wasn't bothered by flying this time. Allan & Ang didn't come this time, so I made sure I had lots of music and some guitar and music magazines to keep me occupied. The pool bar was still there and very similar, but Louis and Maria had left which made it seem just a little different.

The second night, after dinner, I asked my parents if I could stay behind and have another drink to which they agreed as long as I had the money to pay for it myself. I had enough money for just one drink. They went back to the apartment as I stayed for that one drink. I somehow got talking to a couple and her daughter from London at the bar, although I was normally too shy to speak with strangers, they seemed easy to talk too.

They asked me if I would like another drink, I thought it would be rude to refuse, so I accepted and talked with them a little more. Then an Irish couple joined us who were friends of theirs, so I got chatting with them as well. Secretly, it was only the girl I wanted to get to know but I didn't want to make it obvious. The Irish guy asked me if I wanted another drink as he was getting a round in, so again, I agreed out of politeness. After that drink, I went back to the apartment and went to bed before anyone came out looking for me.

The next day we relaxed by the pool, most of which I was plugged into my music in a world of my own. I spotted the girl I liked with her mum by the pool and said hello but we didn't have a proper conversation. That night in the hotel restaurant, one of the waiters said to me, *"That was a cool trick you pulled last night."*

I didn't recall playing any tricks, mum looked at me then asked the waiter what he meant. He said, *"Well, he had a drink with one family, then another family and when he went, one asked the other who he was and neither of them knew. Both families thought he was with the other."* It made me laugh to myself.

We hired a car to go out and find a pretty beach or two as mum loved to see the sea whereas dad was more than happy to just lie in the sun and do nothing except eat, drink and have the occasional dip in the pool. Driving around the island was much more relaxed than the previous years, even the trip up Mount Teide. There was a big part of me that didn't want to go home again, though I was looking forward to Monday and starting my apprenticeship and moving on to the next stage of my life. I was relieved school was out of my life forever, no more homework and I grinned as I played the Alice Cooper song *"Schools Out,"* a lot that week.

Mum gave me a lift to work, expecting to feel suited to the work as I had enjoyed what I'd done at weekends with dad and Chris. I arrived just before eight-thirty as written in the paperwork from the GTA, with my tiny toolbox containing a few spanners and screwdrivers, which dad got for me. I was told that I should have been there at eight, luckily, I had the paperwork to show the start time I was given. A bit later in the morning, the CEO's son-in-law dropped in, he ran the CEO's old family farm. He looked at me and said, *"I know you from somewhere, where do I know you from?"*

"Well, I'm in the Young Farmers club. We did a farm walk at your place about three weeks ago."

Even though I hadn't spoken to him before, he remembered me and said to the manager, *"You have a good young man here, look after him and he will look after you."*

I thought that was nice of him. I learned a lot up until September when I had to start college in Coventry on block release. It wasn't until my first day that I found out I had to travel there and back every day, 25 miles each way, and the start and finish times didn't allow buses and trains to be an option. There was no choice but for Mum to drop me off and pick me up every day as I was still too young to drive.

Although I felt like I was grown up being at work and earning my own money (£50 a week). I was still having to rely on parents to taxi me to and from work and college, which took that feeling of true independence away. My first driving lesson was booked for my birthday, I was motivated to pass quickly. Though it didn't go great, the confidence I had gained from driving tractors around the farm and trucks around the yard went, after stalling that little petrol car five times and going nowhere. Once I finally got it to go and drove it from home to the next village. I had to reverse around the corner and after a few attempts the instructor said, *"Well, this is a new one on me, every time you go to reverse, you turn the steering the wrong way like you're reversing a caravan."*

I said, *"Well, this is the first time I have had to reverse anything without a big trailer on the back when I have to turn the wheel that way."*

All my driving lessons had to be either after work or at weekends, occasionally I could cram a lesson into my lunch break. The limited time off work and college rule was a little challenging at times, especially as I wanted to go on the Young Farmers AGM weekend in Blackpool but it was over a weekend in the middle of my college block and would mean I wouldn't be there on the Friday before or the Monday after. I just phoned in sick to the GTA and let them inform work and college on behalf of me. The weekend was a bit of an eye-opener for me, drinking in the car on the journey, except for the driver that is, then after we checked in to the hotel we headed down to the bar for an hour or two before getting changed to go to the big disco put on at the Winter Gardens. One long boozy party!

Most of the local disco's that I had been to had up to a hundred guests maximum from the same county, this was national and there were thousands of people all having a blast with DJ's from Radio One playing there on Friday and Saturday nights. On Saturday we hit the various pubs around the town before the disco at night. On Sunday, we all went to the pleasure beach to cure any hangovers, though as myself and Dave didn't like any of the rides, except the log flume, we carried on drinking with a different bar to match the others as they went on a different ride. I believe there were some meetings that could have been attended during the day but none of us had time for that! One of the benefits of looking a little older than I was back then was that I never got asked for ID when buying alcohol.

11

Learning To Drive

After the AGM weekend, although it was great fun, there was part of me that was starting to feel like I didn't fit in as I didn't and couldn't drink as much as the others as well as suffering bad hangovers. I considered not drinking but wondered how that would go down with the crowd, as I was teased initially for drinking lager instead of bitter. Wanting a different drink, it seemed, was bad enough but being teetotal would have made me an outsider.

Other than work colleagues whom I never saw outside of work, I didn't have many other friends, as I'd purposefully not kept in contact with most of the people I went to school with. The college lads all lived miles away and stayed in digs together when they were at college, so I was pretty much on the outside looking in there too. And only four of us were HGV anyway, the rest were bus and coach students.

Driving to and from college gave me a lot of driving experience and confidence yet when it came to driving lessons and mock tests, I didn't do quite so well. I think driving the trucks around the yard may not have been helping me at the time but there was no way I was going to stop. Even if the manager's rules were to get your car licence before you can drive the trucks, when I did overtime in the evenings, one of the night shift guys allowed me to drive them.

After five months of driving lessons, my instructor put me in for my test. Although I knew I could drive, it was an exam and my nerves were on a whole new level. A driving licence was the ticket to freedom, no longer relying on my parents to give me lifts, no more calling round friends in Young Farmers to find who was driving and if they were willing to give me a lift and just having the freedom to go anywhere when I felt like it. The nerves got the better of me, I made a few silly mistakes and just caught the curb when doing the reverse park and failed. I felt crushed. I could hardly walk from the driving instructor's car to mum's car. When I got in, she asked, *"How did it go?"*

I believed it wasn't the test that was a failure, it was me. Not feeling like talking, I handed her the result slip instead and let her read it, *"Oh well, you can have another go,"* She said.

I didn't want another go and had wanted to pass the first time. Some of my mates had booked their test for their birthday, turned up with their parents and an old land rover on L plates and passed first time. Then there was me - five months of lessons and I still failed. What made it worse was that I had to go back to work and tell everyone I failed and the same at young farmers that night. Every time the words left my mouth, I felt a little worse about myself and the emphasis on the word *"fail"* felt stronger. I decided whenever my next test was, other than my manager and my parents, I wasn't telling anyone about it. I hated the way I felt and didn't want to experience it again, while I couldn't control the result the tester gave me on the day, I could control who I told about the test. I'd never felt anything like it before and didn't know how to deal with the overwhelming searing pain of having failed inside my body.

My college exams were a little different. The practical exams were based on what the lecturers were observing in the college workshop as opposed to an actual test, which was a lot more comfortable. For the written exam, we were guided by the lecturers on what the examiner wanted to see in our answers and how to word it. We were given many past papers to practice on and I passed all and many with a credit or distinction, but it never felt like I was a success because of the past paper preparation.

At the end of the college year, the four of us that worked on trucks had to do our National Craftsman's certificate tests and were tested at a college in Birmingham. None of us knew what we were going to be tested on so there was no way we could prepare. Not knowing for me did make me feel very nervous about it and questioned my ability to pass it, even though I had passed all other college work.

Sitting in the exam room on D-Day quietly, strangely, just the four of us, feeling distinctly uptight, the assessor spoke up, *"Well now everyone is here, I have some good news and some bad news."*

He carried on talking, *"The bad news is, we can't get access to the workshop we needed to use for your tests, so you haven't got your tests today."*

My mind started going crazy with thoughts about having to come here again and what would be said to work, although it was not my fault, I didn't want anyone to think I had failed it. Oh god.

The assessor continued and asked, *"Do you want the good news? If you do, the good news is that you have all passed anyway. Just don't tell anyone or you may have to come back and re-take them and I may lose my job, even though the tests are very simple and you just have to describe how some things work and identify worn-out components."*

It was a big relief to not fail it but at the same time, it did feel like I'd cheated in some way, despite that we all agreed to not tell our bosses or the GTA that sent us there. On the way back I couldn't help but wonder why we were told many employers viewed this certificate as an indication of being a professional in the field of engineering if all we had to do to get it was show up and agree to keep a secret.

I couldn't help but wish that my driving test had gone the same way. At least I only had a couple of months to go before I had another chance. Passing all of my exams meant I got a pay rise up to £97 a week, which was nice, but it was still a struggle to pay housekeeping to my parents, buy tools to do my job, pay for driving lessons as well as having money left to go out with Young Farmers. I couldn't wait to get all my qualifications and earn the same as the other guys I worked with.

We had another summer family holiday to Tenerife, back to the same resort again. As with previous years, my relaxing ritual was the sun, the pool, a few drinks and being plugged into my music all day. A waiter had taken over the pool bar and for some reason he remembered me from the previous year. Hugo was in his mid-twenties and an islander and his brother Fernando was working alongside him too. As soon as he saw me, he said, laughing, *"Hey amigo, you need a beer? But who is going to pay today?"*

Back at home and back to work, I walked into the office one day and the manager and the two main mechanics on the early and late shift was talking about the other apprentice, who was a year above me. It was one of those conversations I thought I probably shouldn't have heard.

The mechanics were saying that he wasn't pulling his weight and that he needed to try harder, as I stepped back out of the office, I wondered if they talked like that about me too? The manager asked if he was that bad as he thought the other apprentice was doing well and becoming useful. One affirmed that he was, and the other said, *"Well now Alan is here, it is showing him up."*

I wasn't expecting that surprise, but it also felt good to hear, I must be doing something right I thought. I met the young lad who was working on the boss's old farm, it turned out to be Mike, who went to the same schools as me but in a different year and we caught up at a few Young Farmers disco's.

Towards the end of the second year, I wasn't learning as much as I would have liked and one of the night shift guys was trying to coax me to go on nights so he could teach me some different things. I wasn't sure if I wanted to work at night, but the last year had become pretty repetitive and if the next two years were a repeat of that, how would I learn anything more? The GTA said I couldn't work full nights because I was an apprentice. Would I ever be old enough to do anything I wanted? Once again, I found myself stuck. They let one of the night lads go, changed all the shift plans, and wanted one apprentice in from seven till five, and the other from two till twelve, and rotate every other week. The other apprentice wasn't happy as he didn't want to work late, so we asked if he could do the permanent early shift and if I could do the late shift, which was accepted.

I saw this as a good plan for me as I didn't have to be up early, I could learn new valuable stuff between the days and nights. For the first few months, mum was giving me lifts or being in the car while I drove. I was just as nervous as I had been for my first driving test, if not more so on the day. At the end of the test, when he questioned me on the Highway Code, I messed them all up and sighing said, *"I guess I failed again then?"* with a heavy heart.

The instructor said, *"No, you've passed."*

That was such a massive relief I thought, smiling, as I drove myself to Young Farmers that night. Dave said, *"I thought you must have passed as you hadn't called to ask for a lift. I did know you had your test today, as a couple of weeks ago mum came home from a WI meeting saying, "I know when Alan's driving test is," and your mum told everyone there. I guessed as you hadn't said anything yourself, we weren't supposed to know until you passed."*

As good as it felt to be driving at last, it also felt crushing as I had trusted my mum not to tell anyone that I had another driving test booked. Why would she go against my wishes like that, as if my feelings did not matter? Who can I trust if I can't trust my parents? Upsetting questions were flying around in my head. I wanted to ask mum why she told everyone, but I was too scared that my feelings of not being good enough would be confirmed. I couldn't bear that. I wondered why life had to be so hard along with many other questions yet there was no-one I could ask to find out the answers.

Now that my sister and I had both passed our tests, our parents decided to buy us a little car to share, a little black Citroen AX. Well, I say we shared it, that was the intention, I only got to use it about three times in eight months; she hogged it the rest of the time. While I didn't think it was particularly fair, I sensed that I would not gain anything by complaining about it. I got to use dad's van for work and college, though mum still had to give me a lift to the truck yard to pick it up. It seemed a little crazy still needing lifts every day, yet having my license and half a car. If it was my turn to drive to a Young Farmers disco or meeting, then I got to use mum's car, if they weren't going out.

It didn't take long for me to get frustrated with that setup, so when one of my college friends was selling a car, I didn't hesitate and I bought it. I didn't know much about cars but it looked kind of cool. I certainly wasn't aware of checking one over before purchasing. It was a car that stood out; a Mark three Ford Escort, sprayed purple with an RS Turbo styling body kit fitted to it and an XR3i badge. You could say it looked the part but when I pulled up at a set of traffic lights and an XR3i pulled up next me, I wouldn't even consider trying to have a race knowing that my car only had a one-litre Fiesta engine in it, which brought me a little embarrassment and cringe factor driving it at times.

Many of my work colleagues asked me not to park next to them in case it lowered the value of their car. Not to mention my mates at Young Farmers who laughed and refused a lift in my car. It may have not been much, but for me, it gave me a little more freedom, though it was pretty much condemned when it came to its MOT test and I discovered it wasn't safe to be on the road. I left it at work for a week or two until I found someone crazy enough to buy it. I then went to the garage we got the AX from to see if they had anything suitable for me. I left with a Peugeot 309. My friends and family said at least he has a sensible car, so I put an amplifier and big speakers in the back so I could play my rock music very loud.

It also meant I was driving to Young Farmer's events, though it didn't feel the same when you were rationed to only drinking orange juice or Coke. I just wanted to drink there, to make myself feel better somehow, although I still noticed pretty girls at the disco's when I hadn't been drinking. I felt incredibly self-conscious and other than being a chauffeur to return the favours to my friends, I did wonder why I was there. I always felt like none of the girls would be interested in someone like me. Especially when I was out and not drinking, my thoughts would overtake me. What was wrong with me and why I couldn't find a girl willing to go out with me? Was it my looks? Was it just that I didn't know how to talk to them? Was it that I didn't drive a flash car or have some kind of a successful career? Was it that I couldn't dance? Was it just because I was me and just not good enough? It was difficult to go out, relax and be happy when I felt like this.

Maybe if I could dance, I could get a girlfriend, as they always filled the dance floor. When the Young Farmers announced a dance lesson for one of their meetings, I was sold on the idea to go along and see if I could learn. There were some toe-curlingly embarrassing attempts, especially with what seemed like my two left feet. Latin American and ballroom dancing made more sense to me as there was a structure to it which I never felt at a disco. The instructor was also starting a new beginner's class on Friday's and I agreed to go with a few others, surprising both myself and my friends. The first lesson was a repeat of what we had done at the Young Farmers meeting which made it feel a little easier. The instructor's daughter Lucy helped out on Friday. I recognised her from school, and I had sat next to her sometimes on the bus as she was always friendly towards me. She came to the pub with us after the lesson and was very soon a member of the club.

I kept up with the dancing for a few months and earnt some bronze medals before stopping as I didn't have a regular partner to dance with. Lucy kept on coming to Young Farmers and we became very good friends, she also became someone I felt safe enough to open up my darker side too - how I felt about myself, my life and the effects other people had on me as well as girls I liked. I kept this side of myself hidden from most people as it scared me and I assumed it would scare other people away from me even if they did like me, but I was sure many did not in the first place. I felt like some people allowed me to be in their company just to be polite, which felt awful. Many of the Young Farmers thought Lucy and I were seeing each other, or at the least that I fancied her, or she fancied me. Though we were the closest of friends, because we could just be ourselves around each other, we also kept each other's deepest secrets. But did we fancy each other?

12

Hit Like A Ton Of Bricks

We did fancy each other, but alas, not at the same time, so we never got together, even if her dad and my parents would have been happy for us to do so. Allan and Ang introduced my parents to a network marketing business, which they decided to join. I didn't understand it in the beginning as all I saw was mum listening to tapes of what sounded like American people going bananas, while talking to an audience, and reading books about people's personalities. Dad listened to a few tapes but didn't read any books. Mum would often say to me that I would be great in their business once I turned eighteen when it would be legal to join. Some of the tapes were okay and after a while, they were like a fungus, they grew on me, but I refused to read any books as it reminded me too much of school. Those tapes were my first introduction to people with a positive attitude and positive speaking. I was a little anxious about it at first. I often heard the words, *"You can do it,"* which was the polar opposite to what I was used to hearing. After a few months of seeing my parents build their business and attend meetings where they came back in different moods, I decided to go along to a couple and see what it was all about.

After attending one of the business opportunity meetings and I instantly felt that there was no way I could do that. At one of the bigger meetings, some of the more successful people would share their stories and the challenges they faced along the way by way of inspiration for the audience. It didn't change my mind about doing it but while I listened to these people on stage speaking, I wondered if maybe one day I would be on a stage sharing my story. I enjoyed being at this kind of event aside from the business stuff. I came away feeling slightly better without knowing why.

With my eighteenth birthday coming up, I chose to have a bit of a party with just a few friends and no family and have a proper party for my twenty-first. Mum and dad were going away to a weekend business conference and my sister went to stay at her boyfriend's. Not feeling like I fitted in too much at Young Farmers, I only invited a few friends that weren't in the club. Some were girls from school who either worked at pubs I went to or some of the shops in town. Plus a couple of lads that were in different years to me, Mike who worked at the boss' farm, and Kev who was a country lad I knew, that was in Lucy's year at school and hadn't joined Young Farmers.

When the big day came around, I made sure there were drinks and nibbles. Two hours into the party, only about eight people had turned up. Two girls from school who also brought their boyfriends who I didn't know. Mike and Kev, who had bought his girlfriend that I had met only a couple of times. The girls and their boyfriends didn't stay long, telling me they had to go to another party also and wanted to do both. I wasn't sure whether to believe them or not. Before they left, I began to feel a little upset, as some of the people who accepted their invite, didn't show up. I was also feeling down because I had turned the milestone of eighteen and was still without a girlfriend - no matter how many times some girls said they couldn't understand why I was single because I was such a great guy. Every time I heard that line I wondered if they were lying or why they could see things other girls couldn't.

Kev's girlfriend tried to cheer me up and asked if I had good parties previously, so I told her about the farm parties. It led me onto saying what Wiffy had said about coming to the next one and bringing a band along. As soon as I said it, I realised this was the first party I had hosted since he said that, which added to my depressed state, and before I knew it, I was crying like a baby, not knowing why, especially as I was now supposed to be a man, and men don't cry. I just couldn't stop the tears. Nothing anyone said had any effect whatsoever. The only thing that seemed to do anything was alcohol. I just drank and drank and drank until there was no alcohol left. Kev, his girlfriend, and Mike went home and left me with my sorrows. I felt sad that they had left but at the same time, I was relieved that they were not telling me to cheer up, as I didn't know how I could.

I suffered from an almighty hangover the next morning, still feeling bad that Wiffy was not here anymore, it hadn't fully sunk in before last night. It made me realise how unpopular I was and made me think that maybe the Young Farmers should have been invited, as they would probably have come. But with the way I had broken down, I was relieved they had not witnessed that. I think some of them would have seen me as childish and not as a man. I was not sure of what to do with how I felt, other than going to work on Monday and getting on with stuff. I deliberately missed Young Farmer's hockey that Sunday night as I didn't trust the way I felt whilst having a wooden stick in my hands.

It took me a few months to feel like I was getting back to a version of normal, often drinking excessive amounts at the weekends to blot out my grief. I didn't drink during the week in case I lost my driving license on the way to work, plus working late shifts meant I couldn't go to the pub in the evenings.

I joined mum and dad's network marketing business, I still didn't feel I could do it, though I felt it would stop mum talking about it so much. I knew a few people who I thought might be interested and thought if I got someone else to showcase it to them, I wouldn't need to do the bits I was particularly anxious about. Every time I tried to pick up the phone and make a call, I heard a little voice in my head saying, *"I could do it, they said I could at the meetings,"* but there was also a giant towering over me asking me, *"Who do you think you are to think you can do this?"* and it just paralysed me with fear.

I approached some of the Young Farmers on behalf of my parents, I felt less pressure talking about their business as the focus wasn't on me. Some members had poor experiences with network businesses before and me mentioning it was not a good thing for them, which served to strain some of the relationships I had, not because of me or the business itself, but the people who had gotten my friends into it previously.

13

Is This What Love Feels Like?

In previous years I had said no to the skiing trips organised by the Young Farmers, for some unknown reason, this time I found myself agreeing to go. My fear of heights made it a very anxious choice for me and my parents were surprised when I told them. I was advised to get some lessons on the dry slopes before going, whilst others said not to bother because both slopes are completely different. Then there were the special exercises I was supposed to do which felt stupid, so I didn't go to the dry slopes and didn't do the exercises either. I figured if I didn't enjoy it I would go to the pub – my reserve plan that would make it all okay. The trip wasn't until January, to a place in France called Avoriaz, via Geneva in Switzerland.

Not working over the Christmas period and us not having many visitors at home increased my time to worry about sliding down the side of a mountain on two fibreglass sticks and with no brakes! Hearing others skiing from hell stories, such as falling over on ice at the resort and breaking their legs before going anywhere near the slopes probably didn't help much. I didn't express my fears as I thought I might get bullied or teased like when I was in school.

On the Sunday night after hockey practice, just before the trip, it was one of the girls 18th Birthdays so some of us went to the pub to meet up with her and a couple of her friends as they were already in town. The bar staff refused to serve us because they thought we were underage, and we didn't have ID as most of the group at that time were in their mid-twenties. My suggesting to the lad who looked about fifteen that was serving us, that he also needed to be eighteen to serve us, and asking him for ID, may not have helped.

The birthday girl, after a few drinks, let it slip that one of her friends had confided in her that she fancied me. Once I had scraped myself up off the floor at the shock that a girl could fancy me, I asked a little more about her friend and if she would be willing to give me her friend's phone number as her friends had already left. Surprisingly, she did, I wasn't sure which one of her friends it was, not that it worried me as I fancied both of them.

The next evening, I called her friend and asked her if she would like to go out for dinner with me when we got back from skiing. I was as stunned that she agreed to a date as I was to hear she fancied me. Although as soon as I said who I was, she said she was going to kill her friend, so I suspected I wasn't supposed to be told anything. It felt amazing to have a date booked with a girl who had met me and liked me, although I had no idea why and assumed she must have had lots to drink.

Suddenly all of the worries about skiing vanished, all I could think of was seeing this girl and each time I had this warm fuzzy feeling inside which I had never noticed before. Was this what love truly felt like? Having never been in love before I had no clue, and as with many other things, I didn't ask anyone else because I thought I might get teased for never having had a girlfriend.

The week away on the French slopes felt like such a long stretch. My mind was focused on my forthcoming first date. I didn't do too badly with the skiing, no broken bones, though I may have spent much of the time on my butt. I only had one ski keep going down the mountain after I fell over, luckily someone stopped it and stood it up in the snow, so I didn't have to pay for a replacement. I discovered that attempting to ski with a hangover was not a good idea, neither was being the only person without a key for the chalet and the combination of the two was a bit of a nightmare. After two hours of being curled up in a ball on a seat near to the chalet, one of my room-mates came back and let me in. I sent my girl a postcard, but she didn't receive it and found out that she liked cuddly toys, so I got her a little dog on skis. Although I had a good time skiing, I didn't feel I liked it enough to do it again.

We arrived back home late on Friday night and my date was arranged for the following evening. She picked me up and we drove out to one of the country pubs I knew did good food as I often went there with Young

Farmers. Dinner was delicious and I managed to talk more coherently than I thought I would, not too many stumbles over words and even though I knew she fancied me, I was still nervous that she would see the part of me that other girls saw and stayed away from. The part that I didn't know what was wrong with me - I hoped she didn't see it too.

After dinner, we went back to my house for a cup of tea, as my parents were away, I knew the coast was clear. We talked more while we had tea and I gave her the little dog that I had gotten her. Then we kissed. The nerves I had went and that warm fuzzy feeling returned. Although I had kissed a girl before it didn't feel like this one did. I thought my heart was going to beat itself right out of my chest. I had often heard people say when you meet the one you're supposed to be with, you will know. Even if it was love at first sight - was this what they meant? Was this what it felt like?

I asked if she was happy to see me again, and she replied, *"well what do you think?"*

I didn't want to answer that and wondered for a second why she couldn't just say yes or no and keep it simple. I thought it may not go well to say, *"I thought you would be crazy to want to see me again,"* so I said nothing and kissed her instead before asking when she was available as she worked variable shifts at a nursing home. We went out again a few days later, I picked her up this time and we went out for a quiet drink to the same pub. We talked for a while then a couple of the other Young Farmers came in and sat next to us. I'd hoped that none of them would be in that night as I wanted to be alone with her. One of the girls spoke about some health magazine article she had been reading stating that oral sex was more hygienic than kissing. I wanted the ground to swallow me up at that moment, having not talked about anything sexual with my girl and it coming up like that was a little embarrassing and I felt my face flush.

We didn't stay too long after that and we went back to her house. I was a little nervous as her parents were home and I wasn't sure if I was ready to meet them in case, they didn't like me. We had a brief introduction and then she led me straight up to her bedroom. I wasn't expecting meeting them to go quite like that, though it was a bit of a relief not having to chat with them yet. We chatted and kissed and cuddled for a while until she said, *"I think it's time we put a theory to the test don't you?"*

While I was trying to work out what theory she was referring to, she was unbuttoning my jeans. Surprised, having not expected anything to happen between us yet, muttered, *"oh that theory, I think you are right."*

We had a few more dinner and drinks dates and spent time at each other's houses after that.

A couple of weeks into dating my feelings of not being good enough to have a girlfriend started to surface. One evening when I was driving her home, I apologised for not talking enough and felt that at times she would have better conversations with her cuddly toys than she did with me. I knew she could be with pretty much any boy she wanted, and I couldn't work out why she would want to be with me. I didn't feel I had the looks or physique of other guys and I sure didn't have the flashy car or career. What did I have other than I was nice and didn't treat girls like dirt? It seemed like they liked the bad boy types which I refused to be.

Two days later when I called her, she said that I was going to hate her, I wondered what on earth she was talking about. She progressed onto explaining that she couldn't go out with me anymore, it had been great while it lasted, assured me that it wasn't me, it was her and that she was sorry. I didn't hate her but I hated how I felt after that, I hated being single again, I hated that I felt I wasn't good enough for her, I hated myself, but not her. She never said why she ended it or why I would hate her – I was left guessing.

I put down the phone I was using in my parent's room, strode angrily back to my room and kicked the door closed with such force it almost detached it from its hinges. The Iron Maiden poster I had on the back of my door ripped and landed on the floor, I felt enraged at myself for ripping it and not being in control of my actions or feelings. I was home alone, which was probably a good thing as I didn't want to be around any people; not even family. I felt like dying yet I wanted to be in her arms. School didn't teach me how to deal with this kind of thing and neither did college. None of what they taught me felt like it mattered in the real world.

I didn't remember my parents telling me how to deal with these kinds of feelings either. I was at a loss at what to do and I spoke to a few friends who all said in one way or another, *"oh well it happens there are plenty more fish in the sea."* I didn't want a fish. I didn't even want another girl; I wanted her. I felt like I wasn't good enough for her or any girl before we dated, after this rejection, those feelings had multiplied and began to impact my mood in a big way. It was a struggle to get out of bed and to go to work but having grown up with dad having to milk cows on Christmas day, I had been taught a hard work ethic and forced myself to carry on.

Most of my weekends I went out drinking with the Young Farmers and I drank to the point of oblivion but also making myself so ill on both nights that I spent all of the time in between recovering. Being at work sometimes didn't help as I would get easily frustrated and angry when a job didn't go as it should. One colleague was a big well-built guy who played rugby every week and worked as a bouncer on the door at a few of the clubs in town. The manager saw him at the top of the yard one day and asked what he was doing, he said, *"Alan's having a bad day and I'm staying out the way."*

He left me to struggle on. The manager came over and I explained to him about the job *"we"* were doing and how it wasn't going well and that my colleague had just left me to get on with it, which wasn't helping. He didn't ask if everything was okay outside of work or if there was anything else on my mind. He did suggest a few things I could do to get the job back on track which was very useful as I was struggling to think clearly at that time.

I had been noticing the work volume slow down over the past few months, with more and more of the replacement trucks coming through being maintained by the main dealer on fixed price maintenance deals. Some days we would come in to work and just clean the workshop for a few hours before jobs started coming in. The later part of my shift with the night guys was still fairly busy though. I started to wonder about the message from school and what other people had told me before leaving school and starting work; to work hard in school, get a good job and you'll be set for life. It wasn't looking that way to me. I remembered a few people saying that if you have a trade, you'll never be out of work and mum saying that being a mechanic was something to fall back on if being a farmer didn't work out. I wondered if being a mechanic didn't work - what would I fall back on then?

I decided to ask the manager what was going on as it was hard not to notice the work volume reduction, and should I be looking for another job? He said, *"I understand what you mean, we have all noticed it, I can't tell you what to do and it would be a conflict of interests for me to tell you to go and look for another job as I wouldn't want to lose you from this workshop. However, what I will say is that you're still young, you don't have the ties that most of us have and it would probably be a good idea to have a few irons in the fire."*

I thought about his comments for a while when I wasn't interrupted by the upsetting thoughts about not having my girlfriend anymore, even though it had been a couple of months. I spoke to the GTA to get told that they help apprentices find an apprenticeship, but they don't help you get a job at the end of it. I only had a couple of months to go before the end of my third year as an apprentice, then providing I passed, I would then be fully qualified, though I didn't see the promised fourth year to be a refrigeration engineer happening anymore.

I kept an eye on the local paper to see if any mechanics jobs were being advertised and asked the tool dealers if they knew of any openings. I got one interview and the dealer also suggested I call a few local fleets. I said that it was a good idea but that I hated calling people I didn't know; it was a real challenge for me. He just asked if I liked having nothing to do and no money. That prompted me into making up to five calls, if I found a garage looking then I would make another call. I made my five calls and got two interviews booked, I also asked one of the lads in Young Farmers whose uncle had a fleet of trucks if they were looking and I got myself an interview there too. Before I knew it I had four job offers and still didn't know what was going on with my current job. Being in demand like that encouraged a feeling of being invincible and that I would be okay whatever happened.

14

Thank You And Goodbye

Not long after receiving my new job offers, the CEO came over to the workshop, ensuring all staff would attend and after a speech about the business, stories of the past and the company's growth, he dropped his bombshell. They were closing the workshop at the end of June; making us all redundant and all of the trucks would be contract maintained by the main dealers. The guys who had been there for years all said that the quality of service would be different, as when the trucks are with us, they were the priority and that would not be the case elsewhere. The manager spoke up, but it all fell on deaf ears, it was a done deal and I sensed it had been for a while and we were just the last to know. That day showed me that there is little to no loyalty from employers to employees, even family businesses that have been trading for years. It didn't matter if someone was like me who hadn't even finished training yet, or if they had been there over thirty years, the message was the same, *"Goodbye, we don't need or want you anymore, oh and by the way, good luck."*

I queried about the redundancy date being two weeks before I finished college and was assured that course was paid for in full and it was up to my new employer whether they were willing to pay me for that time. I accepted the job with my mate's uncle, who also went to Young Farmers with my former employer, the younger one of the two brothers. He was a bit younger so didn't remember Grampy W much. My theory was that if they were in Young Farmers together, the job may be like the previous workshop. It was due to start in July after my two weeks unpaid at college and a week away in Tenerife.

The new workplace was a much bigger and messier workshop. Two of the boss's sons also ran that side of it and his other son worked in the traffic office. I found it a more daunting job. Working days again did allow me to get back to Young Farmers meetings in the week and go out on Friday, though I had to rise very early to work every Saturday.

One August evening, I went out with Lucy and a couple of other friends for her eighteenth, and ended up in one of the two night clubs in town called Celebrities, although it wasn't my scene. It was my first time there and Lucy introduced me to one of her college friends, her family were originally from Poland although she was born and raised here. We hit it off and arranged to meet up again after a good night kiss, although she was a little nervous and asked if Lucy could join us. We all went for a quiet drink and I got on well again with the friend. Out of the blue, Lucy said, *"Well I can tell you two like each other, are you going to start going out together?"* We were both a little shocked and embarrassed by such a direct question, though it was a question I had in mind. I did like her although she was nothing like my last girlfriend, I thought she may stay with me longer. I said that I would like to go out with her and she agreed.

We went out for dinner the following Saturday, after first picking her up from her house and meeting her dad. A daunting task, although he was easy to talk to which made a difference. We got on well again, but I noticed that I didn't feel the butterflies inside like I did with my last girlfriend. She invited me to a house party at one of her friend's the following night. Despite feeling nervous not knowing anyone else, I said I would go.

My theory of not knowing anyone was found to be correct and most of the night she chatted with her mates and ignored me. It didn't make me feel good and I struggled to get her away to drop her off at home before I could go home and get some sleep before getting up for work in the morning. Most of the evening it had felt like she was more into one of the other guys there, which added onto how bad I felt. I couldn't sleep that night with all sorts of things buzzing around in my head. Why did she invite me if she just wanted to spend time with her friends? Did she like me as much as she said? How close was she to some of the lads in the group? She said they were her people - did that mean they were, and I was not? Was it her way of telling me I wasn't good enough for her? The questions would not stop and as long as they were there, I failed to sleep. I drifted off eventually, though it felt like it was probably just a few minutes before my alarm went off. I had to force myself to get out of bed. I was still on trial at my new job, so I had to and drove there in a half-dead state, luckily my music woke me up a little.

Everyone had a nickname in the workshop and after a few weeks, I discovered that mine was BA. I didn't think that suited me as the only BA I could think of, was BA on the A-Team, and he was the complete opposite of me. I wondered why but thought it easier to go with it than to ask, as I was still getting to know them all.

It felt like I had to work a lot harder there and if I did any overtime, I had to get it signed to be authorised. I was used to just to be able to crack on with my work and no fuss. There were a few perks though, as long as we paid one of the sons in cash, we could fill our cars up with diesel out of the tank they used to fill the trucks up. I found it was cost-effective to ask all three if I could fill up and how much it was at present, as quite often they would all give me a different price, allowing me to get the cheapest offer.

It was good to gain some different experience with the range of vehicles, there were even a few cranes. Being kept busy was a helpful distraction from the endless questions in my head about my girlfriend. I decided I would see her one more time and see how that went and we arranged to go out on the Saturday night and meet up with Lucy, Mike and a couple of other friends plus my girlfriend's friend joined us.

Mike drove us all into town for drinks, all was good, and my girlfriend was quite friendly with me though something felt slightly off with her friend being there. I had no idea what it was and she insisted that everything was okay. She disappeared to the toilet with her friend, in the second pub - I never understood why they had to go in pairs, but it seemed to be the normal thing. After they had been gone for about ten minutes, I was starting to worry there was something wrong, then Lucy read my mind and remarked as to what I was thinking. I hung on a few minutes longer, feeling more uncomfortable as to their whereabouts until Lucy went to the ladies to check up on them and discovered they were not in the toilet and were nowhere to be found in the pub either. Although I had been questioning what was going on between us and how she felt, this caught me by surprise. I truly wasn't good enough for any girl and although it hurt when my first girlfriend ended our relationship, at least she told me and had not just deserted me like this. I drank a lot that night, as I often did when I felt bad as it helped to numb the pain. Lucy and Mike rallied round and did their best to make me feel better but there was nothing they could say that would change my mind on whether I was good enough for a girl.

The next morning, after the effects of the night before had worn off a little, I decided to go and see my date to find out what happened the night before. There was part of me that nudged me to let it all go but I needed to understand why she or anyone could behave like that. The uncertainty of what I would hear filled me with dread, but I had to get an answer. Her dad answered the door and said she was still in bed but welcomed me in to have a cup of tea and he would see if he could wake her.

While he was making the tea he asked what happened the night before, to which I responded that's what I wanted to know and told him what had happened. He said he feared something like that could happen as she had wanted to go out with her friend, but he had forbidden it as her friend was a bad influence and she was only allowed out if she went out with me. I explained that after last night's antics, it was unlikely we would go out again, which didn't surprise him.

When she finally came downstairs, I asked about the night before, not mentioning the conversation with her dad. She said that she liked me and that it was all her friends doing and she was innocent, her friend wanted to go to meet someone else and she didn't think I would like it if she asked me, so they just left. I asked her if she felt that was acceptable and how would she feel if I had done that to her? She answered quietly that she wouldn't like it and it was not okay to leave and not say goodbye. I let it be known then that I knew she was pleasing her dad so she could see her friend and refused to play on her level, feeling annoyance rise in my chest. I bid goodbye and left. Afterwards, I felt a little bad for being so direct, but I didn't want to be used like that again and I knew I wouldn't be able to trust her.

In the same pattern as when my last relationship ended, I drank a lot more and stayed mostly in my room, brooding, with my music for company. It was harvest season on the farms so most of the Young Farmers were busy so when I did venture out, I only saw Mike, Lucy and a couple of her friends, Amy, and Isabelle. I fancied all of them at different times but kept it to myself as I believed I wouldn't be good enough for them anyway, so we remained good friends only.

One day blended into the next, and then into weeks, in a somewhat dreary existence of work, music, sleep, and repeat until the weekend when it was work, music, drink, sleep, then back to work again. When I went out I would see friends and others in happy relationships, laughing together, kissing and hugging and it painfully reminded me of how much I wanted to be like that and how bad it felt to not be good enough for the girls I liked. It was like salt being rubbed into an open wound. The more frustrated and lonely I felt, the more I used alcohol to try and take the feelings away, stuck in a repetitive cycle and the only way I could see it would change would be to get a girlfriend that would stick with me. My close friends were great company but that wasn't the same as having that one girl to have an intimate loving relationship with. I craved that with everything I had.

I was out one night at a country pub, close to where my last girlfriend's friend lived and she just so happened to be there with some of her friends, luckily my ex wasn't with them. After a few games of pool, I glanced over to where she sat and caught her staring at me quite intensely. I wondered what my ex had told her about why we were not together anymore and whether she had accused me of doing something I hadn't. She smiled and winked at me as if she could read my thoughts - maybe she hadn't been told anything bad after all. I carried on playing pool with Mike and Lucy. A couple of times out of the corner of my eye, I spotted her looking at me and flicking her hair away. Each time I thought to myself that if her hair was annoying her that much why hadn't she tied it back. As with any girl, since I was a teenager, she didn't make sense to me. I did notice that the guy she was with at her party wasn't there either.

She got up and began to walk towards me. What should I say if she spoke to me? She said hello and then walked straight past me into the ladies which I hadn't noticed was behind me. When she came out, I said hello back and asked how her boyfriend was. She told me they were no longer together. I invited her to a Young Farmers disco the following evening with our crowd, she smiled and accepted.

There were a few pub stops en route to the disco, and we talked most of the evening, getting a little closer with each drink and by the end of the night we kissed on the dance floor. It helped me to feel a little better about myself, with a girl liking me again, though I did wonder if she would still like me when she wasn't drinking. Would she then find she wasn't into me? I noticed that I'd had these questions with every girl that got close to me - why did I ask them? I figured it was because I was scared they would see that there was something flawed about me like other girls had, which only strengthened my low self-esteem.

We had a second date and after dinner, we talked and kissed on the sofa back at mine. We were still there when dad got up to go to work in the morning. I'm not sure who was more surprised, him to see me awake at that time, me with a girl in our lounge, or us not realising it had got that late. We dated for a while, yet even though she was sticking around I didn't seem to get the butterfly feelings inside like I had previously. Maybe they would develop in time? We saw each other two to three times a week, staying at one another's houses. I didn't feel right at her house though, I'm not sure if it was because their dog slept in her room, which I wasn't used to, as on the farm our dogs were never allowed past the kitchen.

15

Football Is A Joke

My girlfriend's family and friends kept sniggering about a joke connected with football. I found it a little bizarre that they would all burst out laughing when someone just mentioned the word. One night the subject of sport came up and I mentioned that I liked watching rugby but had no interest in football – and there was an uproar! After the laughter died down a little, one of them explained that it wasn't at me or anything I had said but I was the only one not laughing. I felt myself shrinking down and sinking into the floor, the all too familiar feeling of not fitting in. Eventually, I got my girlfriend to explain the football joke a few nights later as we sat in her bedroom. Her older sister shouted from the other room, *"I hope you two are not playing football up there!"* and my girlfriend burst out laughing.

Was the joke about me? When she stopped laughing, she explained that football is like sex - you're either a striker making it happen or a goalkeeper stopping it from happening.

I was relieved to know it wasn't about me, but it didn't justify the laughter it kept getting in my opinion.

As she didn't drive, I was doing extra car journeys and I was still struggling with sleeping and getting up early. I was a few minutes late a few times which did not go down well with one of the boss's sons. I had previously spoken to one of the sons about the possibility that once I was qualified that a pay rise would be given as discussed in my interview. I'd also requested a Saturday off for my girlfriend's 18th birthday as we had something planned and Saturday was overtime anyway. Pay-day arrived the following week and everyone was given their payslip by the foreman except me, he claimed to not know why mine wasn't there and I would have to go to the office and ask. I went to the accounts office and was told I needed to go and see the boss' son. I found him a couple of hours later, now with many questions and thoughts going round my head. He stated that I had a letter with my wage which explained everything, but basically, they could no longer afford to keep employing me. The letter read that my work was not up to the required standard - so why had they kept me on after my three-month trial if I wasn't good enough? But now two months after my trial had ended, I was getting the boot.

To find myself out of work three weeks before Christmas was not good. Being made redundant twice in six months hit the school idea of a job for life out of the ballpark. It did make me feel pretty worthless but was consoled by the thought although I didn't have a job at least I had a girlfriend. I spent a lot of time with her while I was job searching. I played guitar a little too but it didn't feel the same since I heard the comments from Philip's older brother I had a jamming session with, years ago when I'd not been playing long. Him being one of those people who could turn their hands to anything even when they've never done it before. He taught himself to play piano, then after a couple of years switched to playing guitar easily. His comments that did the rounds at Young Farmers, that everyone seemed to know except for me were, *"Oh Alan doesn't have a musical bone in his body, he can't play for shit."* Those were comments from *"a friend"* and cut deeply into my soul. I didn't play for months, if not a year or two after I found out. It didn't stop me listening to my music though - nothing would take that from me.

I found a new job to start in January - one of the jobs I turned down earlier in the year was still available. I had some money saved up so it was kind of like having a month's holiday. Not having to worry about getting up in the morning for work or anything if I had too much to drink the night before was great to start with but got a little tedious towards the end. Although fixing refuse vehicles wasn't what I had in mind when I chose my career path, it was a job and I would be earning again.

The supervisor was also a rocker with long hair and was easy to get along with, but three days into me working there, he had an accident at work. I'm not sure how but he managed to get himself squashed between two vehicles. He did survive but he was off work for ages and so they transferred a manager from another branch to run the workshop, but he had never run a workshop before which for me clearly showed. One conversation I had with him, he said he was struggling to find a job for me to do, so I pointed to one job on the list, a truck with a broken spring. He said that he couldn't let me do that because it was a truck and he felt I was struggling to do car and van jobs within specified times.

My saying that I was a qualified and experienced truck mechanic and had little to no experience with cars and vans seemed to fall on deaf ears. In his mind, you had to be a car mechanic and work up to be a truck mechanic. After three weeks he sacked me with a week's notice. My confidence had already taken a beating with being made redundant twice, now this. It compounded the feelings I had in other areas of my life that I just wasn't good enough and I reached an all-time low. I went home that day feeling very sorry for myself, not knowing what to do next. I told mum what had happened, only for her to say, *"Well maybe dad's transport business will have to vet a van driver or something if you can't keep a job."*

I wasn't expecting her to say anything like that and it was like my mum no longer believed in me either. I shut myself in my room and turned to my music once again. I didn't feel like I wanted another job and to face the fear of being put down or abandoned all over again. I just wanted to drown myself in my music and not have to have anything to do with any people at all.

My girlfriend called me that night as I hadn't rung her for a few days, asking if I loved her as I hadn't called, and she had noticed that I never said those three little words. I was honest and said that I didn't know. *"How can you not know?"* She screamed.

I explained that I didn't know how it felt so how was I to know if I did or not? I told her that I liked her, but that I had heard many people say that when you meet the one you're supposed to be with, you just know and that I didn't feel that. I knew how it felt to have someone say they loved me and not mean it, it hurt and because I did like her I felt it best to be honest. That conversation pretty much killed our relationship and to make myself feel better about it, I thought about the things that I didn't like too much about her and half-convinced myself that I ended it instead of being rejected again.

16

Can I Play With Madness

That weekend dad came home with a potential new job opportunity for me with the guy who was doing his repairs as he had a lot of work built up and was struggling to do it all himself. He wasn't paying very much but it was a job and it meant that I would get to work on dad's trucks. I figured that I'd better take it or I may be forced into becoming a van driver. And, if I did a good job for him then maybe I could transfer onto something that suited me better and be paid more than an apprentice wage.

The first couple of weeks were okay but where I thought working on dad's trucks would be a good thing, it proved to be a little challenging. Not because of the work I was doing with them but more my boss's attitude towards me. He would often speak down to me even when I wasn't working on dad's trucks. One day he came back from an MOT having left me to work alone for most of the day, *"Don't worry you're not the only qualified idiot around, someone applied for a tester's job and where the application form asks for previous experience, it just said he worked for this transport company."*

After working on dad's trucks, my parents would ask how the job had been and if there were any issues they needed to have sorted and so I would talk to them about any concerns. In conversation with my boss, the subject came up and he aggressively told me that even if he was my dad, talking to customers was his role and I just had to do the jobs he told me to do and leave the customers to him. It placed me in a difficult position. I didn't want to be there and didn't feel he was treating me fairly either with his attitude and only paying me £150 for the week however many hours I did, which tended to be fifty-five or over every week.

He did teach me what not to do when it came to customer relations though, after he accidentally ran over one of them with a truck, breaking the customer's leg in multiple places. After that, I made sure I wasn't out in the yard when he was moving trucks around. Over the course of a couple of months what bit of confidence I had as a mechanic deteriorated greatly. I felt like I couldn't even change a wheel without asking if I was doing it correctly. Mechanics was one of the things I had certainty of – I knew I could do it and was good at it until I worked for him. My feeling inadequate became so overwhelming I started to wonder why I was even on the planet. When he bullied me I didn't say anything back because he had a very fiery temper and a very short fuse! I was taught in school to ignore a bully and they will go away.

Out drinking with the Young Farmers one weekend, as I wasn't driving that also meant drinking on the journey into town too. I felt a little down and just wanted to feel numb; to feel nothing. It was normally one of the better events as they hired out a country night club for a private party. I tried to instigate conversations with a few girls but was rejected flat out by all of them. Speaking to Lucy and her boyfriend, I asked him for a cigarette, he refused as I didn't smoke and wasn't about to encourage that habit. Lucy asked me what was up, so I admitted that I wasn't in a great place. I said that I didn't know, but I was thinking of killing someone, killing myself or smoking. She then asked if I was in a place where I could talk about things, I said that I wasn't at all.

Lucy looked at her boyfriend and asked him to give me a fag but he started up again about me not smoking. Lucy knew me quite well, and well enough to know that I needed one in that moment. Reluctantly, he handed one to me. I smoked it with little enjoyment, and it didn't improve my mood, so I continued to knock back the drink, and when I couldn't stomach any more beer I started on Jack Daniels. On the drive home, a wave of further despondency washed over me in my worse for wear state and I felt myself hit an even lower point. Not only was I still wondering why I was here, my thoughts expanded into ideas of suicidal actions. If I were to open the car door right then and jump out in front of a truck, it probably wouldn't matter to anyone. In some ways, I would be doing everyone a favour as I would no longer be a burden on anyone, with me not being up to anyone's expectations.

At that moment, my mate driving, who had no idea of the state of my mind, was looking for another tape to put on to change the music. I wasn't bothered what he put on at that point, I just heard him mutter, *"Oh, I've not heard this for ages."* Then I heard this voice, it was like hearing the tones of an old familiar friend that I had not seen or heard from in years, bringing with it a feeling of safety and connection as it blared out, *"Can I Play With Madness!"* It was the voice of Iron Maiden. Then the music started to play and the lyrics hit me about having the sense to wonder if he is free and himself and having the strength to spit it back in their face. I had to finish listening to this before I jumped out of the car. Then my memory went a little blank and the next thing I was aware of was being back at home and it was the following morning.

Remembering my train of thoughts from the night before scared me - how and why could I think like that but subsequently I was too afraid to tell anyone. My insides felt like they had completely closed-up and I could hardly move. Other than meal times and having to go to work, I spent the whole week locked away in my room listening to my music, wondering why life wasn't fair and what I had done wrong for all these things to be happening to me. The boss hadn't changed over the weekend, not that I expected him to, but it would have been nice. Friends prised me out once for a drink, but I pretty much sat quietly drinking, not feeling comfortable enough to talk about the demons that I was dealing within my own mind.

I didn't think about taking my life that night, nothing sent me spiralling onto that path. I got up late the next morning, walked into the kitchen and my sister asked dad if he'd said anything about Paul to me. I knew a few Paul's so I was confused over which one they were referring to and I wondered what the matter was in the few moments before being told that our cousin Paul, my godmother's eldest son, had shot himself. I was stunned, I didn't know what to say, think or feel. It scared me when it hit home that it could have easily have been me that took my life. I asked if they knew why and apparently, he had been depressed for a long time. What does 'depressed' mean? It wasn't a term I had heard before, they said it was feeling sad and could never be happy.

17

Time To Change

I don't know quite what it was about hearing about Paul, but something shifted within me as I examined how I had been feeling and thinking. I decided that looking for another job was a priority and quite soon found one at the local Subaru dealer who gave me a chance. Although initially my confidence was still low and I hadn't had many dealings with petrol cars, it didn't take me long to get back into myself when I was treated with a little more respect. I looked at what I enjoyed in my life as well as what I didn't and playing hockey with the Young Farmers was a plus and so I joined the local town's hockey club. In my second season, I became captain of the fourth and fifth teams, luckily there weren't many fifths games.

I became more selective as to who I went out with on weekends and where we went. I usually opted to drive on the Friday evening to prevent myself from over drinking as well as making sure I was in a decent state to play a hockey match. On Saturdays, I wouldn't go out until later in the evening also to reduce how much I drank overall. Sometimes I would just have a couple of pints at the clubhouse after hockey and that was it.

Although the fourths regularly only got nine players instead of eleven on their team, seeing some of the young players come up and play senior games from the juniors was amazing. I looked at my guitar that I no longer played. I still loved my rock music and wondered if I would play better and feel inspired again if I got a teacher and some proper lessons. I dropped into the local music store but was quickly distracted from looking for a teacher when I spotted a blue Jackson guitar on the wall. Making a beeline for it, I asked if I could play it. It felt great! I even remembered a few things from years ago. It was a little more than I felt comfortable paying for a guitar so I asked if they would do a trade deal on a BC Rich and they did. Now I had to get lessons to make my investment worthwhile.

I came across an advert for a local teacher in one of the country village papers. Lessons made a big difference although much of the time he was teaching me tunes from his favourite bands instead of the bands that I listened to. He did introduce me to a couple of bands and guitarists that I liked though. It felt much better to know how to play a little more and to be learning from someone who looked at where I was at as a player and taught from there, instead of looking at all the stuff I couldn't do yet. It increased my confidence much quicker this way.

I started to do some car repairs outside of work, which gave me extra money and built my confidence, so it was a win-win situation. It started with friends and neighbours, then friends of theirs, which kept me busy most weekends, which was great. I did a lot for my neighbours Malcolm and Lisa, who bought the house off of the drag racer and Malcolm was encouraging of me to start my own business. Earning some decent extra money was great but I didn't feel I was good enough to get enough work to have my own business. It was definitely something I wanted in my future though.

After all, I was just about to turn twenty-one, the age I could get my truck driving license. To celebrate my twenty-first, we had a party at a local club. Andy, who used to do the long cycle rides with me in primary school, organised the disco as he thrived at hosting them. It was a very messy night from what I remember. Friends, neighbours, and Young Farmers all gathered under one roof in high spirits. One of the youngest Young Farmers decided it would be a good idea to concoct me a special birthday drink. What started off as a Yard of Ale ended up as a liquid mixture of bitter, lager, cider, top-shelf spirits, tabasco sauce, Worcester sauce, and a raw egg. It looked disgusting and tasted worse! I had to balance on a chair at the front of the room with everyone's eyes on me, that alone felt a little uncomfortable as when I was sober I was never the centre of attention and had no desire to be. As I stood there gulping down the horrible slop, a sly thought dawned on me that, the more I spilt, the less I would be forced to drink. I tipped up the glass more than usual so it spilled out both sides of the glass however, I hadn't considered the spillage would go all over my shirt.

Ang was not overly impressed that my shirt was saturated with the disgusting liquid, so she hunted down the lad who gave me the drink and made him give me his shirt to wear until he went home. As the police never bothered the club with it being in the army camp, it often stayed open later than it was supposed to. It was also within walking distance from home and I staggered home at about four in the morning and headed straight to bed. I got up around nine, less than five hours of kip later, and mum was very surprised to see me before lunch. I insisted that I was fine, grabbed some cornflakes for breakfast, ate half of them and then fell off the chair.

I helped Andy out with a lot of disco's he did, mainly with the setting up and stripping down of the gear at the start and end of the night. Each one was its own kind of crazy, as we set up we would see the sunset through the windows on one side of the building and watch it rise the other side as we packed away. There were always drinks firmly in hand from start to finish. Starting with a few beers, progressing onto Jack Daniels until that ran out, then it was shots of Jim Beam until the supplies depleted ending up on the sweet taste of Southern Comfort.

My life felt different a couple of years into working at Subaru and playing hockey. Although I felt like I was as high up the career ladder as I could get there, and I wanted to get back to trucks so I looked for a new challenge. I moved on to do 24-hour roadside breakdown assistance on cars and trucks. I didn't get called out that often at night as they were worried they would wake my parents. It was a family business built up by Charlie, often known as the head man, who started as an agricultural mechanic working out of the back of a van. It was very refreshing to work for someone who treated his staff with respect. As we dealt with breakdowns, we were often referred to locally as, *"Charlie's Angels."* They provided me with my own van, though there were no guarantees that there would be out of hours call outs and they didn't pay any stand-by money but they always said that if we wanted to go out socially, then to do so. I refused to do call-outs on a Saturday night and on a Friday I would go if they called before nine otherwise, I would be in the pub or doing a disco with Andy.

I gained my truck license with them after a week's intensive course, which they paid for providing I didn't leave straight away and go to drive for dad. I thought getting my car license was hard, but this was harder. There were two of us doing the course that week and on that Friday morning, the instructor said we both did well and expected us to both pass. We both failed. I failed another two after that, for giving a cyclist too much room, then not giving a cyclist enough room, then for not overtaking a cyclist fast enough. Each time I had the same examiner, but on the fourth test I had a different guy and he passed me. Then I got my license to drive a truck with a trailer on the back, which I passed on my third attempt, again the third test was with a different examiner to the previous two. It was disheartening to fail as many times with something I knew I was capable of and wanted to do. Just like when I sat my regular driving test, if I saw the examiner mark his clipboard I went to pieces, assuming the worst and made lots of mistakes after that point. Even if he was just scribbling his pen to make sure that it worked, in my mind, it determined my failing.

Being on emergency call out for the police to go and pick up all of the mangled vehicles after crashes was an interesting experience and made me stop and consider the way people, including myself, drive, especially when one of the bloody vehicle collisions was the same make and model as my own car or one of my friends. I used to drive at two speeds, fast and stop. This along with driving trucks and being aware that there are many blind spots that a truck driver has and they just wouldn't see my car, slowed me down a lot. Being on call did mess up a few things though, it made it difficult for hockey, especially trying to organise the team as captain, so I stepped back from that position and just played as often as I could. It also complicated guitar lessons as I often got called out before I got to my lesson. Then my teacher went off travelling to America on an opportunity that came up suddenly. He was due to fly out the day of one of my lessons. That day was the same day that the planes went into the world trade centre on 9/11. I was relieved to hear he wasn't on one of those planes but at the same time, it annoyed me a little, as the search was on to find another teacher.

I saw an ad in a guitar magazine, for a week's intensive guitar teaching at the Academy of Contemporary Music in Guildford. I booked the week off and went for it. There were some amazingly talented players taking part and others that were not far off beginners, which is where I decided I fitted. One of the teachers I had was Pete Friesen who played with the Almighty when I saw them at Donington and supported Iron Maiden and Metallica. He had cut his hair short, but I could tell it was the same man. To learn from him gave me a real buzz and during one of the classes, he used some Alice Cooper and Almighty tunes to teach us how to do things.

After the lesson, I waited behind to ask him about the Almighty and let him know that I had seen him play with them. He then gave me a half-hour private lesson focused on showing me some of the Almighty tunes. We chatted and he explained how he had left Alice Cooper to join them and when they split, he went back to Alice. The Almighty decided to reform for another album, but he said he couldn't leave Alice again. I asked about his intro at Donington and the Wayne's World comment. He laughed and said that he was in Alice's band when they filmed Wayne's World and he was in the movie. He also surprised me when he shared how all of the guys were scared stiff for Donington; it was their biggest gig and they didn't know how well they would go down and were scared they would be the next, *"Bad news"* (Rick Mayall's band) that were booed off in less than sixty seconds at the Metallica gig at Milton Keynes. However, they believed in themselves more and that was his best gig with them.

I asked what made him want to become a rock star? He expressed that whilst growing up, he looked at his dad's generation who worked, got tired, retired broke and didn't get a chance to live or see the world - he felt he had nothing to lose and played non-stop, practising for hours and hours a day, every day, especially when he didn't feel like it. I asked what he would have done if it hadn't worked out. He said he'd probably have had to get a job or some shit, but he wasn't willing to let that be an option.

I realised after talking with him that these rock stars were not gods on a pedestal as I had previously thought, they were normal human beings with a strong passion for what they did and were willing to put the hours and hours of practice in for years, which I had not. I knew I probably wouldn't be a rock star after that but I did have something inside of me that wanted to open people's minds.

While I was away, I got a text from mum to say that Gran E had died, there wasn't anything I could do so not to come home but stay and enjoy myself. Unlike when my grandfathers passed, I knew what it meant, it was sad though but as she said, there was nothing I could do, so I buried my sadness and carried on.

When I got back, I went looking for a new guitar teacher and the guitar shop put me in touch with a teacher in town who shared the same kind of musical tastes as me. His abilities blew my mind, not just in how he played, but I could take along any cd, and band, playing at any speed and after listening to it a couple of times, he'd say, *"this is how you play it."* Whether it was blasting out thrash metal rhythms from Metallica, their solos or the galloping lead harmonies from Iron Maiden - I lost count of the times I watched him, truly mesmerised and wondering how the hell do you do that? He was able to show me what both guitarists were doing at the same time and was impressive and inspiring. He would break down all the parts in a way that I could understand and made it much easier for me to implement, otherwise I would be daunted by it and it seemed unachievable for me.

Occasionally I would bump into my teacher while I was out on a Saturday night. One night I saw him in the Chicago Rock Cafe, which had become a bit of a regular thing for me, Mike, and a couple of other friends. I was just chatting to him when Mike alerted my attention to a girl across the room and asked if she used to be in Young Farmers? As soon as I looked up, I knew it was her straight away. She only went to a few meetings, but I did get quite close to her and hadn't seen her for years. I went over and spoke to her, although I could tell she had been drinking she seemed pleased to see me and gave me her phone number and we arranged a date.

We dated for about six months, but she suffered from anxiety attacks, which seemed to complicate things and she seemed to go hot and cold on me. I couldn't always tell how much she liked me. She came on holiday with my family to Tenerife. A couple of weeks after we got back, she went on a canal barge holiday with her family for a week, although she was gone for two weeks which seemed a little strange. When she finally returned home and called me, I asked her where she had been for the second week. She said that she was on the barge for two weeks, the first with her parents and the second week with her ex-boyfriend as she never stopped loving him. I said that she was supposed to be my girlfriend and he was supposed to be her ex, but she couldn't understand why I was upset as she went on holiday with me too. I felt like she had no respect for me or our relationship and neither truly mattered to her. I'd been helping her do a lot of work around her house and on her car, none of it had been appreciated.

Suddenly, I felt like I was going down the same path I had in the past and it scared me. I didn't want to go there again. I remembered how it felt to be in dark places and that terrified me. I was still too afraid to share with anyone about all that and how bad it had been for me. If other people knew, would they want to lock me up in a padded cell? Give me a strait-jacket and fill me with drugs as they did in some of the movies? Or just tell me to man-up and get over it as worse things happen at sea? Or to stop being so over-dramatic? I didn't want to find out what the outcome could be.

I had a day off work; feeling down and for some reason, I felt inspired with an idea and walked into the careers office and asked if they had any information on fixing boats in Barbados. They hadn't but they offered me some information about working holidays in Australia and New Zealand. Although I knew a few people who had travelled there, I was aware that there were a lot of snakes and sharks and things in those far countries that eat people, so could I go there? But then if I was eaten by a shark it wouldn't be my decision, it would be an act of God and would be easier for my family.

I thought my parents would try to stop me going or tell me I was crazy having heard similar desires from me before with wanting to play guitar and go to rock concerts. But when I said I was considering it, they said it was a great idea and to go and do it. Mum said she wished she had the chance to go when she was younger but there weren't such options back then, and it would be good for me to have an adventure. An adventure? I thought. You have no idea what's in my head; no-one did, which was probably for the best, so yes, we can call it an adventure.

18

Runaway

I made the decision to go in August and I planned to leave in October but then Rachel, Allan & Ang's daughter, had met a guy in New Zealand while she was travelling and was due to have a baby and marry him here in England not long after I would have been due to leave. I decided to delay my trip until after their wedding, which gave me the chance to save up some extra money also, though it meant getting another job as I had already quit the one I'd been doing. I landed a nice easy job doing some MOT's and juggled that with a job behind the bar at the Chicago Rock Cafe in town. Although I only worked two to three nights there as well as the garage, it was pretty tiring.

Serving behind the bar one night, as I went from customer to customer, a familiar voice chirped up, *"What the bloody hell are you doing there?"*

It was Andy. We got to catch up later in the evening when it was a bit quieter. I told him of my travel plans and that I was starting in Perth and going on from there. He advised me to start in Brisbane and then he'd come with me as he had family there. I was sold on that idea, as I was very nervous about going alone.

I had a lot to organise to make the trip happen, which seemed to take ages. A colleague's girlfriend was a travel agent that specialises in out of the ordinary trips. I went to see her and got my flights booked plus overnight stays along the way until I landed in Australia. I called Andy and said that my flights were booked and gave him the dates. Once that was done, everything else just fell into place. At Rachel's wedding, I spoke to her about travels and she assured me that I'd love it as everyone is so friendly and at the hostels, everyone is in the same situation so they become friends easily. One of her friends said that the best way was to go alone but that for me still seemed very daunting. I was pleased Andy said he would come out with me, even if he could only stay a few weeks.

A few weeks before I was due to go I decided to have a leaving party to celebrate and just in case I didn't come back, as there was a big part of me that had no desire to do so. The only people that couldn't attend were the people I worked with at Chicago's, Andy, as he was DJ at the club in town, and my godmother. Rather than spend half the night at the bar, I printed off a little drink voucher for all my guests to have a drink on me and put a hundred pounds behind the bar.

The following weekend I had arranged to go into town with Andy and his girlfriend. When he said he couldn't come, I initially thought he meant for a drink, but he meant that he couldn't come to Australia at the same time as me. We met up for a few drinks and ended up in Chicago's. I was given a free bottle of bubbly off the manager and my choice of one song to be played. It had to be Metallica, *"Wherever I May Roam,"* which felt very fitting at that moment in time. Although he played *'Unforgiven'* instead, which was a bit sad although still a great tune. Andy's girlfriend said she was sick, so he had to leave early, just as I had ordered another round. So I was there alone with three drinks lined up. We were all supposed to be going home together so I didn't know how I was getting home now.

A regular at the bar and also a very generous guy when it came to buying drinks for the staff, came up to say hello and asked why I had three drinks when I was sitting alone. I explained my situation to him, offered him one whilst I finished my drink then had Andy's and had another couple of drinks with him before it closed, and everyone got kicked out. I still hadn't figured out my method of getting home, so the regular customer offered to let me crash on his sofa if I wanted? As the taxi queue was extremely long and a few people were fighting over them, I thought it was a better idea than the alternative six-mile walk home. I still had the bottle of bubbly with me which I was going to give to mum as it wasn't my kind of drink. When we got to his place, we had a night-cap before my memory went very hazy as I started to fall asleep on the sofa. The next thing I knew it was morning and I woke up feeling very strange, so left as soon as I could. It wasn't the normal hangover feeling, as far as alcohol effects were concerned, I felt fine but instead I felt disoriented and wasn't sure where I was or what had happened and my bottle of bubbly was empty.

That time seemed like a mystery to me and I felt I may be judged for staying with some random guy in his house and by claiming to not know what had happened. That fear of what other people could think of me scared me nearly as much as my fears of what he could have done if anything. I consoled myself with thinking that surely if anything had happened in that missing period of time, I would remember. As with so many things, I did my usual trick and I buried it and hid my fears from everyone.

A few days later I went to see my godmother for a cup of tea as she had to miss my party night. As we chatted about my plans, as with mum, she assumed I was going for the adventure. I didn't have the strength to say I was running away or what I was running from. Our conversation reminded her of when her sons had travelled to Australia. As we talked about how time flew by, she started to reminisce about their trips and as she realised it was five years since Paul had taken his life, she started to cry. I didn't know what to say or that there was anything I could do, so I just sat there and let her feel whatever she was feeling.

As she sobbed, I saw something in her eyes that I had never seen in anyone before. To try to put that into words I can only describe it as a pain that may never heal and never go away. I felt sad that there was nothing I could do to take that away for her. At the same time, within my mind, I had a vision of my parents crying in the same way at their kitchen table if I had taken my life. I knew in that moment, that no matter how hard life was or what I ever went through, there was no way I could pass that sort of excruciating pain onto my parents.

I promised to go and see her whenever I got home, as I did with many other people. The big day arrived, and mum and dad took me to London Heathrow Airport. I was still very nervous, as I'd not been away anywhere on my own before. Now I was going half-way around the world and not coming home for a year, maybe longer. No half measures for me! We ate breakfast at the airport and said our goodbyes. As I walked away towards the security gates, feeling anxious, I felt my eyes welling up with tears and

I dared not look back and let them see me cry. I had almost two hours to wait before I could board the plane, the point of no return. After that plane door closed I knew that I couldn't change my mind. I had to fly.

19

Down Under

After a three-day stopover in Singapore, I landed in a rainy Brisbane, which was refreshing after the plane's air conditioning and the hot and sweaty humidity of Singapore. I got a taxi to my hostel where I had booked to stay for the first seven nights, other than that, my only plan was to be in New Zealand for Christmas and spend time with James at Rachel's home. I wandered around for a few days exploring the city and doing some of the tourist stuff. I chose not to go to Steve Irwin's Australia zoo with all the reptiles and creepy crawly creatures. I was sharing a three-bed dorm room with an Indian guy in his late forties (who was looking for a house so he and his family could emigrate there) and the person in the third bed changed every night. So much for the, *"Everyone's in the same situation and you make friends easily,"* idea.

I tried to get bar work in the city, but I needed a hospitality license which I didn't have, I still had enough money in the bank so decided that a job could wait for a while. I visited Movie World and SeaWorld, then fancied some chilled time on the beach. The hostel receptionist was a friendly long-haired surfer guy who called everyone *"mate,"* like a true Aussie, recommended Surfers Paradise on the Gold Coast. I paid it a visit after catching up with Andy's aunt and uncle for dinner and passing on a delivery for his mum.

Surfers got me, the week before I could easily have boarded a plane and returned home or gone onto somewhere else. The people at the next hostel were like a family and suddenly I felt switched on and understood what travelling was all about. My roommate was a guitarist and had bought an old acoustic from a charity shop and he let me play it whenever I wanted. We discussed why he had gone travelling - he claimed that he was a mess and had to smoke a couple of spliffs and have a few drinks before he felt able to go and have a quiet drink with his mates.

Although I was never into smoking or spliffs, I could relate to having to do things to feel comfortable in order to go out - I wouldn't go to a pub on my own unless I knew for sure my mates were going to be there. It was like a security blanket for me. Yet here I was on the other side of the world on my own and knowing no-one, that was a deep thought for being in a sober state at the time. Maybe it was what my old neighbour Lisa meant when she said, *"To make sure you take time to sit back and reflect on what you're doing."*

Two weeks later my bank balance had depleted rapidly due to partying and alcohol. I could not get a garage job either as I had no tools with me and wasn't willing to buy any here. Instead, I found a farming job application company and after a week of their farm training course and they sent you out to farms on work placements as they had national connections. On the bus journey, I sat next to a German lad who was going to the same place. As we got out into the countryside, I asked how much farm work he'd done before, to which he replied that he hadn't even set foot on a farm before. I said, *"You see those funny looking black and white horses over in that field?"*

He said, *"Yes."*

"Well, they are cows mate." I laughed.

I sat back in my seat imagining that I must be going to the Australian version of the Billy Crystal movie *"City Slickers"* - it certainly felt like it. Even more so after a couple of days at the training farm, with the farmer instructing us how to drive a tractor, how to feed cows, ride horses, motorbikes and then teaching us to round up cattle on horseback and riding motorbikes. It was amazing to be back living on a farm again; it brought back fond childhood memories. I still missed the space, the fresh air, and the freedom.

At the end of my course, I went to work on a farm in New South Wales doing lots of driving in tractors that were controlled by satellites and repairing stuff in the workshop. I found I got on better with the Aussies who lived and worked there better than the other backpackers working there. We all left together, as one of them had a car and we all chipped in with the fuel money to drive across to Byron Bay but from there I let them go on without me. I needed my own space to run wild and free wherever I felt called to be not where they chose to go. I noticed low moods had crept in when I was with them. I toured up the East Coast to Cairns and Cape Tribulation by bus, stopping off in Noosa Heads, Fraser Island, and Airlie Beach along the way.

From Airlie beach, I gained my open water scuba diving certification, although the skills tests with removing my mask and taking my air regulator out underwater scared me, I did it.

Scuba diving was another world. As hand signals are the only communication, size, looks, and body shape didn't matter and all that mattered was keeping an eye on each other and our air gauges and breathing. It was liberating to leave the nonsense of the world above on the surface. The course included a three day live-aboard trip out to the outer Whitsunday Islands on the Barrier reef, three days of eating, sleeping and diving, cut off from the world on land. On the last dive, I was coming down with a cold and couldn't equalise my ears and had to stay above five meters in depth or it was just too painful. There was also a strong current, so we just drifted as we explored, but as we came to the end of the dive, we surfaced to find there was no boat. We not only could not see our boat, but we also could not see any boat, anywhere. A couple of other divers surfaced, and they were perplexed as to where the boat was too. We didn't think it would have left without us and we chatted about what to do and decided to swim along the surface against the current back in the direction we had come from underwater. It was hard going but once we got closer to the end of the cliffs to our right we could see around into the next bay and there in view was the boat. The current was much stronger than the instructors had expected, and we'd travelled twice as far as we should have done. We were all relieved to get back on board. It also made me realise how small the world could be – I was taking part in a dive course in Australia with a guy who lived in the next town to me back in the UK!

I continued up the coast to Cairns and discovered that to be another party town that depleted my bank account and one of my favourite bars was Jono's Blues bar for the live music. It was an oasis of the love of music, life and being able to freely express yourself. Sunday nights boasted the gong show, where members of the audience could get up and perform whatever they wanted. I longed to participate and play live guitar, but I dared not get up. I spoke to Jono one night and he suggested for me to pick a song I could play, then join his band on stage and he would perform the vocals. It was still a daunting idea but I went for it and opted for *"Sunshine of your love"* by Cream. I wanted to run off of the stage but I felt I'd be laughed at, my body started to shake with thoughts that I was getting it wrong, so I turned down the volume on the guitar so no-one could hear me if I messed it up. Jono noticed he couldn't hear the guitar through the monitor and turned it up. A three-minute song felt like a lifetime, but it felt good to finally be on stage with a band, that was a big achievement. I didn't win the prize of a diving trip, but I didn't get booed off stage, which was a huge relief.

I headed off to the next farm which was a cattle station in the outback, three hours from Alice Springs. I settled there for three months despite the station owner not treating staff well, often speaking down to them, including me. I felt myself going down a rabbit hole as it reminded me of old experiences. It being an extremely remote location was a big benefit, off of the water mains, so all of the cattle were watered by a pump from a borehole, most with a diesel motor and a couple with an old windmill. Every two days I had to go out and make sure all the cattle had water, that the motors were fuelled up and the tanks were not overflowing. That process would take all day - ten to twelve hours. That time out working solo gave me time and space to think, talk and listen to myself properly.

It was out there that I realised I had failed and had failed before I had even left the Country. My plan was drastically flawed. I had gone abroad to run away and get as far away from all of my problems as I could. Now I realised that I had taken my problems with me, just as I had my backpack, as part of my luggage was my beliefs, my fears and my insecurities. I could not run away from them. With that mind movie playing out of my parents crying at the kitchen table, I knew I had to find a way to deal with myself. I thought about those books that I refused to read with the network marketing business.

I contemplated the remainder of my trip and how I could better use the experience and my time alone. I headed over to Perth and spent a couple of weeks with some friends of friends. I enquired at the immigration department to see what I would need to do if I wanted to stay there. I had two options - I could cancel the rest of my travel plans and work as a mechanic for six months which would allow me to stay. Or keep my plans, go back to England and work as a mechanic for a year and then I would still have enough points to come back and stay. They suggested that I should take some time and on a sheet of paper, write on one side the reasons for being in Australia and on the reverse side the reasons for being in England.

I spent a day on the beach doing exactly that, in the end, I had about fifty reasons for being in Australia and just three for England: family, close friends and no snakes. Those three were a very heavyweight on the balance between the two. I wondered what the balance would look like if I were to do it again on British terrain. The next stop was a flight over to New Zealand to meet up with James and to travel. The Kiwi Experience bus was certainly interesting. It felt good to see familiar faces and to be on holiday with James again after a long break. It proved to be a most strange experience wearing shorts and having a barbecue on Christmas Day though. Jumping off the back of a car ferry that had been converted into a party boat, straight into the freezing cold sea at midnight to see the New Year in, was almost up there with weird escapades! Even though I was with James and Rachel over Christmas who were pretty much family to me, I still harboured feelings of not fitting in there, it was almost like I was an outsider looking in on my own life. Was there something wrong with me to be still feeling like this? I kept it to myself as I thought that by me saying how I felt, I would be judged a little and appear ungrateful, after all, I'd been kindly invited into their home as a guest for Christmas where I could have easily been sat in a hostel alone. I also missed my own family a little, as it was my first Christmas away from them.

I took a radical approach in an attempt to cure my fear of heights by facing the fear head-on by putting myself forward for a skydive. It was a great scenic flight until an idiot opened the door and said I had to get out.

Hanging off the edge of the plane, only held on to the instructor with the parachute by three little clips I suddenly felt very unsafe and vulnerable and desperately wanted to get back into the safety of the plane. The instructor told me to stick my tongue out for the camera, to which my whole body froze as if to say, *"Fuck that"* I don't want to do this anymore. But I reasoned that if I backed out, the girl with the other instructor who couldn't jump until we did, would then reveal to everyone in the hostel and on the Kiwi Experience bus how she couldn't jump because I was too scared. That was almost as scary a thought.

The choice was taken out of my hands as my instructor leaned forward, then none of us were in the plane any longer and we were free-falling. The exhilarating high that Dave Mustane sings about in the Megadeth song, *"High-Speed Dirt,"* wasn't there for me – I felt more like, *"Say a prayer for me now because I'm going to die."* I had never been so relieved to be standing up on my own two feet, in a field in the middle of nowhere. Mum and dad were not overly impressed when I sent them a text with the message of, *"Oops I just fell out of an aeroplane,"* dad replied asking if I was okay? Not even considering I may have been skydiving - but then he did receive the message at about four in the morning.

Early into the New Year, I headed back to Australia, stopping off at Sydney, Melbourne, and Tasmania. I had been communicating with the family that I was going to stay with, in Tasmania for months. I'd be working for them for a few hours a day in exchange for bed and food. Steve and Bronny with their two children Kate and Nick, lived in the countryside with a few animals and a garage business. I soon felt like I was part of the family there.

They were also musical and had guitars, drums, and a piano. They knew my taste in music in advance and mentioned to me a friend of theirs, Mike Tramp, who sang in White Lion and Freak of Nature before doing his own solo records. I got to meet Mike a couple of times, the first time he popped in I got him to sign one of my White Lion CD's and then the next day he returned to give me two of his solo CD's, both also signed. That for me was a true act of kindness and made me feel special. He was good friends with Lars Ulrich of Metallica, both originating from Denmark. Mike seemed very down to earth and humble for a rock star, reminding me of when I met Pete Friesen. I felt sad to leave there, probably even more so than leaving home in the first place, as I didn't know if I would ever make it back although I wanted to. I promised to go back for Steve's fiftieth birthday, which was still a few years away.

After Tasmania, all that remained was a few days in Melbourne for the Grand Prix and then I'd fly home four days early via Thailand. I texted mum to see if I could wind her up as she didn't fall for my skydive prank. I said that I had been stopped by the police for drunk driving Mike Tramp's ute on the way back from a rodeo and they were going to deport me. Though there was some truth in the message, I hadn't been stopped by the police and I certainly wasn't being deported.

20

The Tasmanian Devil

My flight out of Melbourne was delayed by a few hours as the plane was broken and they were awaiting parts from Sydney; that sounded reassuring! I missed my overnight stay in Bangkok and it left me with just a few hours to wander around the city, get some food and a drink or ten. Going from Melbourne to Bangkok's hot sun, then onto a cold, snowy London was a big shock to the system! Luckily my parents greeted me with a big winter coat for me to wear.

Reflecting on my trip; it had been the most mind and heart-opening experience I'd had at that time in my life. I was relaxed and happy, although I knew I had to find a job, a car and get back into life at home again. After a year of not being answerable to anyone, just friends I made along the way and not staying anywhere longer than three months, I felt like I was ready to settle down. Especially after being back living with my parents for a couple of weeks. Back to being asked where I was going, who I would be going with and when I was going to be home? Inside I was screaming out, *"I am twenty-seven for crying out loud - not seven. Do you need to know all this?"* I decided I had to get my own place within a year. I couldn't do it straight away as I had some travel debts to pay off and had depleted my savings more than I had anticipated and didn't want to rent. I got a job working nights as a truck mechanic as I had been before and only a few months down the line I had been promoted, so I cleared my debts and started to save money again.

I worked four, sometimes five nights a week and at the weekends I went out with my mates. My search to meet a girlfriend was still important to me, yet when I was out I still didn't seem to meet any. Even after travelling, I didn't find it any easier to meet and get to know girls, I never knew what to say, or if I had something to say I would get tongue-tied and any words that did come out my mouth sounded a little like the

Tasmanian Devil cartoon character. I didn't know why or how to change, or if it were possible, as it had always been a challenge for me and the age-old feelings of not being good enough or unattractive to girls was firmly fixed in my head. There was a solution known as internet dating and I warmed to the idea of being able to chat first, so a girl could get to know me and who I was on the inside, and see that I wasn't the kind of bad boy that my girlfriends used to always get hurt by and complain about. I was always the one who picked up the pieces and wiped their tears away yet they wouldn't date me, even though they all said that I was a good guy. To say it still confused me was an understatement.

After a lot of online chatting and one or two dates, I had gotten quite close to an Asian girl who was studying hotel management in Belgium. She wasn't going back to her family in the summer holidays so she came to England so we could meet. We got on well, with some things in common and still had a lot to talk about. I went over to Belgium in the Autumn and she came to me for Christmas. We spent time together over a few more weekends and holidays and started to look at what the possibilities were for further developing our relationship.

I bought my house in January 2005 and I'd had to move to a different town to make it possible though it was the same travelling distance from work as my parent's house.

She was very keen to get married but I had a few reservations as we still didn't know each other that well. I felt like I was ready to settle down though and in part, I was fearful that if I didn't marry her, then I may never meet another girl who was willing to settle down with me. We explored all the different options for a visa, with her not being a UK resident.

We both wanted a family with two children and to have our own businesses as well as to travel, despite sharing a few cultural and language differences and personality clashes at times. Having never had much success with girls and my sometimes crippling self-confidence issues, I believed this could be my best chance of a successful relationship.

On my next trip to Belgium, we both went to speak to the British Embassy and organised for her to get her visa to allow her into the UK as my fiancée and part of the rules were that we had to be married within three months of the visa being issued. I felt we were forced into rushing a little and I spoke to my parents who said, *"You won't get to know her any better just going there, or her coming here for a few weekends a year,"* and, *"Don't worry, if it doesn't work out divorce is much cheaper than it used to be."* I still had their support with it.

Not long before she was due to emigrate, a concerned Andy came round to ask me if I had considered that maybe I was making a mistake and that she may be just doing it to get a British passport. I told him that I didn't feel that was the case, even though it had crossed my mind and that I was well aware of the risks and thanked him for his concerns.

She moved over to the UK to be with me in August 2005, and we were married in October. A couple of weeks before the wedding I had some doubts, but my family reassured me that it was just cold feet and everyone got that before the big day. One of my stipulations was that her parents had to attend our wedding; firstly, to see their daughter get married and also so that they could meet me. If I had a daughter, I wouldn't want her to marry someone I hadn't met. They didn't speak a word of English and we didn't speak a word of their language, so she had to translate everything. Her dad would talk for about five minutes and after asking her what he said and she would just say, *"Oh nothing."* Much of the time I had to communicate with them using scuba diving hand signals and facial expressions.

We had discussed her dad's father of the bride's speech many times and she insisted that he knew what he was going to say. It was a different story on our actual wedding day and when that moment arrived, she told him to stand up and I could tell that he hadn't a clue what was going on. I asked my wife to tell her dad to say thank you and sit down, which he did. She spent most of our wedding reception evening in her parent's bedroom with them and I had to track her down so that we could have our first dance. I thought it was very strange that a girl who wanted to spend her life with me disappeared on our wedding day but figured her parents were getting old and being unable to speak English, they may have needed some extra assistance.

My new wife didn't look too impressed when the DJ announced our first dance as Iron Maiden's, *"Phantom of the Opera."* She didn't realise it was to wind up a couple of friends before cutting over to Extreme's, *"More Than Words."*

21

Married Life

The first year of our marriage wasn't too bad but it was a far cry from the *"wedded bliss"* dream that society speaks about. It had its challenges as the visa rules prevented her from being able to work or have any kind of income. Everything I suggested that she do to get out of the house and make friends, or even just to occupy her time and mind, she dismissed as a bad idea. I was still working nights which felt like it caused a little tension between us on top of that, so I changed my job so that I could work days and we could see each other more. That change created a different kind of stress as I was earning less money each month, although I earned enough to cover our living expenses.

I thought it may be worth having a business we could do together, though as she had no real qualifications or work experience to draw on, we decided on her working for mum and dad's network marketing. I still didn't feel it was for me but I felt it would do her some good and help her to create a new life outside of the home. After a few meetings and appointments, she lost any interest she had and pulled away from it. One of the meetings we had attended showcased a couple from Ireland speaking. He had been expelled from school at fifteen and had to work in a butcher's shop. Although I didn't want to do that business he inspired me to explore different possibilities as well as reading those books I'd kept putting off and learning new things.

Still filled with the hopes and dreams I came back from travelling with; I started my own business in my spare time, fixing cars to build a second income with a view to it becoming a full-time business. I found that while I was good at doing the actual job and had the skills when it came to business growth, marketing and sales I wasn't very good and had a lot to learn as all the jobs I'd ever had, someone else always took care of all of that. One of my clients was a business coach and after a few months of not having many clients, I decided to hire him.

My wife wasn't overly happy about me investing in my business, she thought it was a waste of my money, as I was paying out for income protection insurance and house insurances. She tried to control how I should spend my money and how she wanted things in my house to be. Each different item came with a hefty price tag that she was not willing to contribute towards as it was my house.

Her comments began to drag me down. A few times I was told that I needed to buy a garden shed to get changed in after work so that my work clothes didn't pollute her clean air in the house. It never went down well when I reminded her that I was already paying for the house, so I was entitled to get changed in there. Then followed remarks from her about how I wasn't successful as I wasn't earning enough, then she would go on to criticising how I would do the housework and that I wasn't doing it properly. There were all sorts of other negative things as to why I wasn't a good enough husband and she compared me to her friends' husbands. Each comment on its own wasn't too detrimental but the build-up of nasty criticism overtime was hurtful and knocked my self-esteem a bit more. In some ways, it felt like I was back in school hearing the cruel taunts or back working for the guy who told me off for talking to dad about his trucks.

The second-year things started to change as her mum's health was starting to fade so I said she could go over and spend some time with her mum. She went over for three months, and I joined her for the last two weeks. When I went out, I had to meet her sister for the first time at the airport and she took me to where my wife was. After dinner together, numerous taxis arrived so we could meet up with their cousins who took us to sleep at their house for a few hours. Afterwards, we embarked on a long car journey to the city where my wife's parents lived. The following day, after about six hours of driving and various phone calls to keep them updated on their mum's condition, there were some deafening screeches from the back seat of the car. Their mum had died with still another hour's drive to go.

Once we got there I realised just how different our cultures were. When a loved one passed no-one was allowed to sleep until the deceased had been buried – which would happen two days later, just what I wanted to hear after only three hours sleep in the last twenty-seven hours! It was exhausting. After all of the funeral proceedings were done, we left her family and went our own way, with a few days in another city before flying home together. I had missed her but not her negative comments, which now started getting worse as she saw it as my fault that she didn't get to spend enough time with her mum or to see her that last time. I thought it was unfair to be blamed for it as the time she didn't get to spend with her mum was a result of her decisions not to stay at home and her parents' decision to have their children raised by nannies and childminders.

We had a few differences in the way we wanted things to be if we were to have a family. I believed the best carer for young children would be their mother as they would have a stronger bond with her than anyone else. She wanted to have a child-minder or nanny because being a mum would be hard work that she wouldn't be paid for. As with any other disagreement or a different point of view, she was right and I was wrong and if I didn't see things her way, I hadn't listened or was stupid.

During the next year, her comments worsened as did the way I felt about myself, she had an amazing ability to flip things over and make me feel like the results of her decisions and actions were somehow my fault. She told me that her cousins had twins by IVF and asked how I felt about doing the same so she only had to get pregnant once. I refused point-blank. I didn't believe in treatment unless we had been trying to get her pregnant for a few years unsuccessfully, then it could be an option but not when we hadn't tried. She went back to her country again for another three months to see her family and because she wanted to do a massage therapy course that would be cheaper for her to learn in her country than in England. Although I suggested she would be better to get certified here as it would be recognised and easier to get insurance.

I went with her for the first two weeks then left her there. While we were there she suggested that we had sexual health tests, initially, I thought I'd prefer to get them done at home, but as I hadn't ever had one before, decided it may not be a bad idea. She wanted to make sure everything was okay with both of us before she tried to get pregnant. I thought and hoped that maybe if we had children, she would be happier and not give me such a hard time.

My business outside of my full-time job had increased my income and I was working towards being in that business full time. She was also working full time, as the visa now allowed her to do so. Most of the time she was away from home. I had suspicions of some of the stories about her work that she told me but with no proof, I didn't say too much. I was suspicious of the way she would only ever look for a job via her own ethnic community and it was always a job away that forced her to be away from home, that paid cash in hand and provided accommodation for her.

It was the fourth year of our marriage and she had yet another trip to her home country; this time to see her sister and father again and catch up with some friends. I didn't go on this trip as I had too much on with work and business, as well as never being able to see the parts of her country I wanted to see. Though secretly, I just wanted peace and quiet. The day before she left we had unprotected sex which was the first time in our marriage.

About a month after she had left, she told me that she was pregnant - just like that. First time? Wow! When we were talking a month later she revealed to me that the baby had no heart rate and the doctors recommended that the pregnancy be terminated. She decided that was best and the procedure had been done the day before. I didn't know how to process my feelings or even what the feelings were. It just felt like someone had ripped my insides out. I did my best to support her though, I didn't know what I could do for her being so far apart. The following two weeks I felt like things couldn't possibly get worse, but I got taken by surprise, to say the least. To start with, she told me that she was sick and that it would have been passed onto me, so I needed to go to the doctor. I enquired as to what my doctor would need to test for and what the symptoms would be. She said she had to ask the doctor there and she would let me know. When she did get back to me, she told me that she had Syphilis. That didn't sound good as I knew that I had been faithful, so I went to the local clinic the next day and had all the tests done and the results were all clear. The doctor that gave me the results confirmed that unless my wife had some kind of blood transfusion with infected blood, she had been having an affair. The only thing that seemed strange, was that they didn't check my sperm as they did at the hospital in her country the previous year.

That same week whilst searching for a flash drive that I had mislaid, I found one of her notebooks. It was all written in her language, which I didn't understand aside from a few words such as, hotel names, men's names and prices. Along with notepad were hundreds of condoms, different to the ones we had been using, newspaper clippings of massage parlour adverts, bank statements in her name showing deposits of hundreds of pounds from around three different cities; all hundreds of miles away from the place she had informed me she was working as a waitress. I got her little book translated; in a way I was hoping that it wasn't what I was suspecting but the translation just made me feel worse. Not only did it confirm my suspicions, but it was also very explicit. I couldn't help but think this was probably where her Syphilis came from. My heart just sank to the ground and filled me with thousands of unanswered questions. How could she do this to me? Why would she do this? How could this be going on without me knowing? Why couldn't she talk to me? What should I do now? How can I talk to anyone about this?

In all my failed relationships never had I been treated in such a way as this.

22

I Want Answers

The questions went on and on and I did not receive any real answers! I felt so much shame for myself and the situation I was in. I did feel like somehow I had failed even if I didn't know how, where or when, and that ending our marriage would be the best thing now.

I wasn't sure how to bring this up either on text message or voice calls, so I just kept communication to a minimum. I spoke to a family law solicitor to see where I stood legally and told my family that we were going through some challenging times, which they had suspected anyway, I just didn't go into any of the details.

I followed the advice of the solicitor as I didn't know how to handle this for myself or who I could talk to without being criticised or judged. The solicitor advised me not to mention what I had found or what I was thinking of until she was back home as she may just never come back which would make divorce or moving on very difficult. I had the day off work to collect her from the airport and planned to get things out in the open that day. I didn't feel comfortable talking about it all in the car so I waited until we got home. I'm sure the atmosphere was so tight it could have been cut with a rusty butter knife.

When we arrived home, I said that we needed to talk. I told her my test results were clear and I wanted to know where she got Syphilis from? She tried to tell me she must have gotten it from a towel or a toilet seat which I refused to believe. She couldn't give me a proper answer, so I moved on to all of the other stuff. She tried to explain that the condoms she was looking after for a friend who had now left the country. That reminded me of high school when friends got caught with cigarettes, they would get another friend to phone their parents and say they were theirs instead. All her explanations just appeared to be made up and pretty crazy. I just couldn't believe them. It was probably not helped by me no longer trusting anything that she said. After a while, she just said that it would be better that she didn't speak. How were we to move forward if we didn't talk?

I didn't feel I had any options left and I threatened her with divorce if she didn't tell me the truth. I went out for a walk and when I came back, I said that I needed the truth even if she felt I wouldn't like it. She still refused to talk, so I got the divorce papers served. I felt kind of bad doing this on the day she got back, but things would only have gotten worse and worse if I left it any longer.

The next day I got home to find her in tears. She had read the divorce papers and reality was setting in; she knew I wasn't messing around. She said that she had spoken with some of her friends and they recommended that she tell me the truth. She said that she had been working in a friend's office taking calls from the working girls and taking notes for the boss. She didn't feel she could tell me as she didn't think my family would approve. The money she had lent to a friend who was paying her back bit by bit, when she got the money together. She still couldn't explain the Syphilis or the condoms. She then admitted that she was never even pregnant while she was away. The hospital we went to in her country was an IVF clinic and she wanted me to think I had got her pregnant naturally before she went, then would get herself pregnant with a multiple birth from the clinic instead as she had spoken about wanting to do. That completely destroyed any chance of me trusting her again. I felt like I was in an impossible position.

I felt that I was having to choose between continuing with the divorce and with the possibility that she could come back one day with multiple children and saying that they were mine and that I needed to pay for them, which may cause issues with a new partner if I had moved on by that point. And the other side was to let her get herself pregnant, knowing there was a strong chance that our relationship still wouldn't last, but knowing that if it ended and I moved on, I'd be a single dad with however many kids. This would be easier for a new partner to understand than the other option. It was a big decision to make from a low place, as I was mentally and emotionally drained.

I decided on the second option, I needed to have some kind of certainty in my own mind as to what she was likely to do. Two months later she went away for 2 ½ months and came back pregnant with twins. The hospital called us one day to discuss some results and we had to go to the clinic where I had my STI check done. The doctor we spoke to that day said they had picked up a trace of Syphilis, which would always be present in her body and wanted to make sure that she had been treated for it. This made me question everything even more and made me feel like she had been tested and had treatment before going to have the IVF done the first time. Any inkling of trust I had left for her was completely gone after that.

Though the pregnancy went well, they had to perform an emergency C section early as the second baby was no longer growing. It was a worrying time in so many ways. Both babies were born healthy and needed to stay in special care for almost three weeks. During this period, their mum only went to visit them twice! The nurses at the hospital were starting to get concerned as I was going in every day and they said that if she didn't start spending time with the babies to bond with them, they would have to get social services involved. I didn't like the idea of that so the next day I took her in to see them before I went to work and left her there for the day. She did start to bond a little and the hospital was happy to let the children come home with us once they were stronger.

Life with newborn twins would be challenging at the best of times, but we had all of the other stuff hanging over us too, it was far from easy. Four months later my neighbours informed me that it had been noticed that my wife was going out and leaving the children at home alone for a few hours at a time and was I aware of it? I was not and certainly didn't agree with her doing so. I talked with her and let her know that she had been seeing doing it and that it must never happen again. She just said that they were her kids and she would raise them however she wanted to. I said that she may raise them how she wanted to as long as they were not being put at risk and that she stayed within the laws of this country. If she was caught leaving them again, social services would be informed, and they had the power to take our children off us if they felt it best for their well-being. It was most disturbing and upsetting.

Just a month later, I came home from work to find that she was out. I was initially relieved to find that she had taken the children with her this time. I didn't know where they were and as I walked around the house, I noticed other things weren't there either, the laptop, baby swings, milk bottles, steriliser, and more of the baby's items. I called her but there was no answer. Then I called the two friends of hers that I actually knew but they knew nothing either. The neighbours said that they saw her load the car up, cramming in as much stuff as possible, with the kids screaming in the back before she drove off. They didn't know where she went to either. I called the police and reported them missing and said that I wasn't sure about her mental health at this time, as I had been told she was leaving our children just six months old at the time at home alone. They said they would look into it and after half an hour, the police said that they were aware of their location and that they were safe and well. They wouldn't say where she was, only that I needed to get some legal advice. I did speak to the solicitor but there wasn't much they could do at that time other than hire a private investigator. It was an awful time as I longed to have my children back and know for certain that they were safe.

Two weeks later my wife called me and said she did what she did to teach me a lesson and she wouldn't tell me where they were or when I could see the kids and just laughed at me down the phone. I couldn't see anything funny at all about our situation, my blood was boiling inside. After a while, she agreed to bring our children over to meet me in town. When we met, she said it was better for us to live apart as we would get more money off of the government that way and that she didn't want any money off me. They were her kids and that she would take care of them on her own. Then I started to receive calls from the CSA saying that I had not been paying her any maintenance. I agreed to pay what I could afford, but it was never enough for her as she believed I could afford more with a full-time job and my part-time business, despite being shown my financial situation a few times with bank statements and accounts.

23

Reality Hits

It was a very tense time between the two of us for a long time. The first Christmas after she left, she returned to the family home. I didn't want her there, but I was so desperate to spend time with my kids I felt like I didn't have a choice. She said that she had returned home to see if I had become a better husband. Also that she had to have the kids on her own for the last few weeks and it was my turn to do everything for them. Even though I said that I was coming down with a bad cold and the children were likely to catch it, she still insisted that I did everything for them. I gave the children their Christmas presents on Christmas morning after breakfast following my family's tradition, though their mum said they couldn't have her presents until the afternoon. I found that to be a little strange, as they were so young, then later in the morning, she wrapped up the gifts they'd been given from the refuge they were staying at and gave them the same presents again and said they were from her. I couldn't believe what I was seeing. I thought that it was pretty low, and she would have no chance of doing things like that when they were older and wiser.

After ten days, they were gone again, with both children coughing and spluttering from the cold germs that they caught off of me and I could only assume that I had not become a better husband, not that I cared about that anymore, as there was no way I would have her back. A couple of months later she filed for divorce listing a few reasons that were either lies or just comical. I spoke with my solicitor who said that while I could contest it, as I still wanted to be divorced from her, it would be better for everyone and more cost-effective to let it go through as it was.

I followed my solicitor's advice in that mediation would be good for us in the hope that we could talk through a few things and come up with a deal and not need too much solicitor input. Going through mediation was painful, as I had to sit there listening to her telling lots of lies to the mediator, though I just kept believing that the truth would come out in the end. We both had to provide three months' worth of bank accounts for every account we had, including all debts. For the second meeting, she turned up with one bank statement and said she didn't need to provide any more because I was the bad guy. The mediator explained again that we both had to provide information and that she was impartial. The following meeting she brought along details of one account, but after I questioned her about other accounts, she got angry with me and said that her money was her own and she wanted half of the equity in the house - not realising it was in negative equity at the time.

The divorce went through and I got to see my children regularly, although the collection and drop off was still tense as I didn't want any arguments in front of the children as they were innocent parties in the mess we had created. Every time that I went to collect or drop off the children, I dreaded it as I didn't know what she was going to come out with next – she was very unpredictable. It was very clear to me that I was Satan in her eyes, and just my breathing and existing alone should have been a criminal offence.

It was hard work holding down a full-time job, building a business in the evenings and on Saturdays and then having the twins on Saturday night and Sunday. Almost a year after she left, my monthly salary went out within twenty-four hours on legal fees and child maintenance. Out of frustration and determination, I left my full-time job to focus on my business. My business was turning over a few thousand more than the gross salary from my full-time job so I felt like I had nothing to lose.

Over the next few months, it did get a little easier. There was a reduction in her late-night phone calls in which she would complain that she couldn't get the children to sleep and it was because my blood was in their veins. Though every time I picked them up I would get a lecture on how I had to take care of them and another one when I dropped them off to say that I hadn't looked after them properly in some way. The bond between myself and my children kept getting stronger. I think it had always been there since I was the one that spent more time with them when they were in hospital before coming home. Looking back on this time it's like I was some kind of zombie or an extra in the movie of my own life and I was just watching it unfold, wondering what was going on and who stole the script. My body was there but much of the time I was not.

Things went well for a few months. I started dating a new lady, which felt amazing and for the first time in a long time I felt that a woman could see me; the man inside of my body. This only lasted a few months as she felt she needed to spend more time with her own children, as well as trying to work out what went wrong between her and her husband. Although their marriage was over long before we met, they still had things to sort out. That hurt as it reminded me of my feelings of not being good enough that I had been fighting for years and even though I had done nothing wrong, it still felt the same.

At the same time, the guy who was renting my house out had died, having breached the contract we had and having his girlfriend living there without telling me or the council. The reality of my situation hit home, I was struggling financially and I felt like I had failed as a husband, a father and was currently failing as a business owner. I couldn't afford to keep my house but I couldn't afford to sell it or rent it out either. Kneeling on my living room floor I sobbed, not knowing which way to turn, contemplating running away again and starting a new life in New Zealand. The lyrics of the music I was listening to made me stop and think, I felt like I'd been hit by an express train. As Mike Tramp sang *"Better Off,"* it resonated deeply, and I felt like he was singing about my kids in the future if I didn't make some changes in my life. No-one else could do it for me. I just had no idea how!

24

Reflections, Realisations and Growth

As I fantasised about running away, I recalled the reasons for my trip to Australia and how I took my problems with me. It wouldn't solve or change anything and would mean that my kids would grow up without their dad in their lives and they were the innocent parties in this mess. They deserved better than that, they deserved a dad who was there for them and one they could depend on. The thought of letting them down and not being that dad hurt. The following week I had a meeting scheduled with a lady who was a coach who had been recommended to me by a friend of mine.

As we talked, I knew I had to hire her for myself. I couldn't afford her fees but I also knew I couldn't afford to fail my children. Working together I discovered that I had been burying and suppressing emotions for many years and only seeing the things in my life that I didn't like or were not the way I wanted them to be. My investment in myself and personal development began to sky-rocket, nothing was going to hold me back. I attended weekend seminars with Tony Robbins and T Harv Ecker, as well as my weekly life coaching sessions and monthly business coaching sessions; I read dozens of books and listened to educational cd's.

In working with my coach, I found that many of the things I had believed for years were not true and just a story that I'd created in my head; a powerless victim story, after all if something was outside of my control and had nothing to do with me, how could I do anything about it? I was looking for the world outside of me to change to match how I believed it should be. One of the questions both of my coaches and Tony Robbins asked, *"Was what I had done to contribute to the situation?"* It turned out to be a very powerful question although my initial answer was nothing and that she or he, someone or something did this to me. The more I learned about the human mind, emotions, and behaviour, the more I learned about myself and how in fact, I had actually done a lot to contribute to the situation.

One of the events I attended encouraged me to look at how my life was now and how it would be in five or ten-years-time if I changed nothing; that was painful. I had visions of both of my children being on drugs, involved with prostitution and all sorts. And then I had to come back to the present and see how life could be different in five, ten and twenty years having made inspired changes. That was much more pleasant to envision as both of my children were looking up to me and telling me how I had inspired them to go for their dreams.

So how did I contribute to the collapse of my marriage? Firstly, the communication at the beginning between the two of us was in no way deep enough or specific enough to know if we were in any way a good match to spend a life together. I didn't communicate how I felt for two reasons; one being my intense fear of rejection and not being good enough, and two, that often I just didn't know how to pinpoint how I was feeling let alone put it into words to articulate myself clearly. Often when she would ask me if I could or would do things, I would agree, go ahead and get stuff done.

When I was bullied either in work or at school, I would not speak up or stand up for myself, sometimes that was driven by the fear of being physically beaten or making it worse as well as not wanting to turn into a bully myself. If I didn't say that a person's comments were hurtful either to the person saying them or to ask for help from someone else, how would it stop? Also, a bully may comment on one occasion but each time that I replayed that scenario in my head over and over again, aside from the initial event, it was down to me. When a girl ended a relationship with me, I chose to tell myself that it was because I wasn't good enough, where actually she was saying that she knew she wasn't a match for me and set me free to be available for a girl that was.

Was it my fault the farm sold? Was it because I didn't matter? No and no, but it was me that created the story in my head that it was centred around me and it happened to me, not taking into account any of my family or what they wanted or needed to do for them. I also see that it was a blessing in disguise as many farmers were struggling and not many were happy. I was reminded of this as I wrote this chapter in January and subject to the constantly changing weather, there were flooded fields all around and farmers everywhere were unable to get onto the fields to plant their winter crops and many of the seed suppliers quickly sold out their stocks of spring seed. They needed the fields to dry out in time for planting so that the crops could grow in time for harvest.

Ultimately, I came to realise that I am responsible for the feeling *'farm'* in myself, where every thought is a seed or a weed. The more I focus on the things that make me feel bad, the worse I will feel. I get to choose what crops to plant and good thoughts will provide the crops I desire. Sure, other people and life may throw rotten seeds into my field, but it is down to me to remove the wild seeds and weeds. If I keep planting lemon seeds and expecting a fantastic crop of apples, I will always feel that I'm not good enough, yet the crop and harvest will never change until I deal with the root or seeds I'm planting. Also, if I do find rotten seeds or crops, I am a lot more careful where I throw them, and some people have yet to learn how to deal with the rotten stuff.

I used to complain about the bullshit life kept throwing at me but, on the farm bullshit is natural fertiliser to encourage the crops to grow ready for harvest. The bullshit life has thrown at me has allowed me to grow. Once I moved out from under it and stopped drowning in the mire. I would often tell myself that I didn't fit in, now I just look at myself and say that I need to be outstanding in my field, even if that means standing alone. Though I am never alone, not when I know I have loyal friends who have been with me in my darkest times and those that believed in me even when I didn't believe in myself.

That belief I had about girls and women just liking the bad boys I found out to also be a BS story that I had repeatedly told myself instead of taking the time and effort to learn. Yes, some do like a bad boy, but it's more the traits of confidence and the excitement and uncertainty that he portrays that some women are attracted to. Yet when he is called to take responsibility for things or to be emotionally available, he disappears out of sight. When did two bridesmaids ever say to each other, *"I'm so pleased our friend is marrying this guy - he's such an ass?"*

Women also like a man who is nice, who will listen to her like a true friend without judgement or agenda and to be their rock amidst their emotional storm, but too much of the nice guy and she gets bored as he gets predictable. They are attracted to a man who has the courage to be a gentlemanly leader and take responsibility for things, and stands up to her when needed, after all, how can she believe he will stand up for her if he will not stand up to her?

The challenge for a man is in learning which of these guys to be for his woman and at which times, as she desires all three in one man. I used to think I had to be one or the other. I had only ever been a nice guy and I didn't want to be a bad boy who hurt girls and I had no idea that the leader even existed.

These are a few examples of many beliefs that I have re-framed and replanted. I saw David Hyner speak, having interviewed many successful people in many areas from business and sport and other celebrities. I always remembered what he said about interviewing Olympic athlete Kriss Akabussi, *"So Kris, how does it feel to have everyone look up to you?"*

To which he replied, *"That's where everyone goes wrong, they look up to successful people, instead of looking into them, to find what drives them, what makes them tick and where their passion comes from."*

For many years I looked up to Iron Maiden and Metallica but from that moment on, I looked into them and respected them and their music even more. After seeing an interview with James Hetfield of Metallica on where his music came from, one of the things he said was that it gave him a voice that he wouldn't have anyway. I asked myself, *"What do I have in me that I don't have a voice for?"* I could talk about events in my life quite easily but how I felt about them was another thing altogether. Within an hour, I had the lyrics to the following songs. *"Day by Day,"* was inspired by the day I came home to find my children were gone and *"I'm not your enemy,"* was inspired by the things I was struggling to communicate to my children's mum.

Day by Day

Came home that fateful night,
taken from me far from sight
no-one heard me scream no-one heard my call
jumping up and down screaming at the wall
I had to find you somehow, some way!
I could not wait to watch you dance and play

Minute by minute, hour by hour, day by day,
this nightmare had to pass it can't stay
minute by minute, hour by hour, day by day.

I missed your touch, I missed your smiles,
missed your laughs, even your cry my little child
couldn't get you out my heart or out my head.
everyday I would see your empty beds.
So hard to take the pain,
very near drove me insane.

Minute by minute, hour by hour, day by day,
this nightmare had to pass it can't stay
minute by minute, hour by hour, day by day.

My heart full of sadness and even rage,
I found my faith, things would surely change.
my feelings and emotions locked in a cage
but still my love for you would never stray
faith told me you'd be with me some day.

Minute by minute, hour by hour, day by day,
this nightmare had to pass it can't stay
minute by minute, hour by hour, day by day.

I am not your enemy

It was wrong from the start,
we came from worlds apart,
a vague idea it could be right,
required communication so far from sight,
 it was more like a business deal
than any love that could be real,

We all have broken dreams
but life isn't as bad as it seems
poor choices from the past,
some things are not meant to last
many conditions to your love
don't you see you're blessed from above

All you see is someone to blame,
and expect me to think the same,
is this the way you want it to be?
I am not your enemy.

Why not learn from what's been and gone,
it's time for us to get up and move along,
it doesn't matter what was said and done
no-one is right and no-one is wrong,

All you see is someone to blame,
and expect me to think the same,
will you ever even see?
I am not your enemy.

25

Energy

As Albert Einstein famously quoted about energy, *"Educating myself about energies has been a big lesson for me and how both masculine and feminine energies are within me as well as every other person on the planet in much of the same way that each magnet has a North and a South Pole."*

My desire to be liked by everyone and attractive to everyone had me trying to be 50% masculine and 50% feminine. I also found that I was much more attracted to more feminine women with my core energy being masculine but a woman who is more feminine in her energy will be more attracted to more masculine than I was at that time, even if it's subconscious So I found that I was making myself less attractive by being something I was not.

A woman who is more masculine in her core will also be more attracted to a more feminine male. Energy is not specific to gender or sexuality, as men being attracted to women and vice versa is the most common and I am using that match as an example. A strongly feminine energy lady will be able to feel with her intuition in no time when a man is not being fully authentic with her. If he is more feminine in his core yet tries to be masculine as it is how many men get conditioned to be.

Since learning more about myself I have connected with some amazing women, beautiful inside and out, yet like me, they have been through a lot before getting to the point that we connected.

For two years I dated a Norwegian nurse with her either coming to me for a short period of time or myself going there. She opened my mind and heart to what was possible, although the limited awareness I had of energies before we met, I had thought I was right in the middle, yet she would often say that she loved how masculine I was. I was still struggling to understand energy, but I appreciated her insight as that was where I wanted to be. We had been looking at the possibilities of living together but it had to be right for both of us, my children and her son. It ended when it became clear that despite loving each other we were heading into different directions in life. We are still good friends today and she is happy with the love of her life.

Although there was a part of me that still wanted love after that, I was happy to just be me and the kids. However, during a challenge to get a clear relationship vision in a personal development online singles group, I got to know a lady in America. This connection told me a lot about unconditional love and love being about what you give not what you get. Though we never got to meet it felt amazing and there was a real buzz between us. At one point she went quiet for a few days, then I received a voice message from her, almost in tears because she had found a lump on one of her breasts. She was also in a position where the week before she had lost her job and her employer had been paying her medical insurance.

Having had cancer twice before, she was not in a good place and I wished I could do something to help but being on the other side of the world and financially broke, my options were limited. I wondered what it would be like and what I would do if she had to have a breast removed before coming over and the only answer I could come up with was to love her anyway, if not more so, for her courage and bravery. I learned what it meant to hold space for someone to feel. I learned that although I may need to be in the same room to hold her hand, I could hold her heart from anywhere. One of her close friends offered to marry her then and let her be on his insurance. Having no real options and two children to support, it is what she did. A few months later she messaged me to say she was cancer- free, I have not heard from her since.

I took some time out of dating after that, I had a lot to process and to decide if I was even interested in being in a relationship after that. I deeply questioned the old saying *"love hurts,"* and as I looked back on my dating history I could easily buy into that idea (note that not all my dating history is within this book, I've not included any that could cross other people's boundaries by sharing).

Then on a deeper level, what do I and many other parents do when their child falls over or has a bump with no damage done? *"Would you like daddy or mummy to kiss that better for you?"* Their bump gets kissed, they get a hug and they go off to play again as if nothing happened. That hug and kiss is love, love doesn't hurt, love that heals. So why can relationships be so painful I wondered? If it's not love that hurts? Rejection hurts, unmet expectations hurt, unwanted or unexpected behaviours hurt, disrespect hurts, broken trust hurts, and crossed boundaries hurt, but not love. All these things make it feel like love hurts, where it is the feeling of the loss of love that hurts. Love is about giving, all these things come from looking at what is being received.

While going through all of these reflections, I remembered my conversation with Pete Friesen and how I wanted to make a difference yet being uncertain of the way. I thought about the difference coaching had made for me, so I booked myself onto a weekend coaching course in London. I had a chiropractic appointment the same day that I booked it. My chiropractor has also had some toxic relationships and came out of the other side and happily married an American lady. In talking about our journeys, he mentioned energy and spiritual healing. I didn't know what these were, and I wanted to find out and he gave me the contact details for the healer that he saw and decided to book an appointment.

A social media friend had also been talking about energy healing and spiritual things, I couldn't help but wonder if some of my challenges were energy or spirit related as they cannot be seen. She recommended that I connect with a couple of her friends, Luke and Eugina, who were putting on a retreat in a few weeks-time. I talked to them and it sounded like something I needed to do.

I had my first energy and spiritual healing session. I don't know what happened. The lights were dark, there was some relaxing native American music playing and it seemed like I was asleep without being asleep; what I do know is I felt good afterwards. The healer asked what the connection with London was? I said that I didn't know as I hated the place, but I was going there for a coaching course in a few weeks. She told me that London was going to be very good for me. I asked how she knew, she just said that energy never lies.

131

The coaching course was very good indeed. In going through the processes and questions taught with the other delegates, I found some very interesting stories I had been telling myself over and over again since I was a child. My junior school teacher that scared the life out of me with the story and meaning I had given to that, was that women are scary. The story now says that she may have scared the five-year-old me, but she doesn't scare me now and neither do any other women. What I heard my dad say as a small child, *"Children should be seen and not heard,"* my mind translated that as I should be seen and not heard. And I should not talk to strangers, yet all of my friends were strangers before I got to know them, so sometimes a stranger is just a friend I haven't met yet.

I found that I had a strong belief about loss, as my grandfather was taken from me, some of my friends were taken out of my life, the family farm, my future, and my identity were taken from me, jobs, and girlfriends had gone from my life. There was no point going for my dreams and desires, or even to make friends as they would only be taken from my life and that would be painful.

With all these things connected, when it came to approaching a girl I fancied when I was in my teens or twenties, my eyes would see her and I knew that I would like to know her but my programming always said that I can't talk to strangers, that I should be seen and not heard and if I did get to know her, she would be taken out of my life, as well as the natural fear of rejection that everyone has. Realising this, I could then see how just saying hello would cause me to freeze to the spot and unable to speak. It felt very freeing to understand this and it was as if a lot of weight had been lifted from me.

A month later I headed off to Essex, for the retreat with Luke & Eugina, although I had seen the briefing information and chatted with Luke on the phone so he could make sure I was a good fit. I wasn't sure what to expect which did make me feel a little nervous. Knowing it was going to be a week of a vegan diet also made me feel a little anxious as I like my meat much more than veg. I knew that other than two of the facilitators, Luke and Sia, and the cook who would be ducking in and out between cooking, that I was the only man there along with four women. During the five days, we went through native American prayers and rituals and shaman rituals. During a freestyle dance activity, we were told to pick a song, and then later we found out that we had to dance to it alone. I picked *"Sweet Child O'Mine,"* by Guns n Roses, which felt like it went on for a lifetime! There was just one rule with the dance; if Luke didn't think we were playing full out, we would have to do it again and try harder. At the end of my song I was exhausted and relieved that I didn't have to repeat it.

The intention behind everything we did was of letting go of limitations from the past, learning how to express ourselves and to process and release emotions in ways that worked for us. There were many tears, from everyone as they made their own breakthroughs and let go of past fears and shame. Well, all except me that is, I was the only one who didn't cry even though I had talked about some of the painful events I had experienced. The guided meditations that we practised, mostly sent me to sleep and Luke woke me up about six times during one of them.

On day three, during the late afternoon/early evening Shaman ceremony we practised, I didn't feel at all comfortable. I just couldn't relax into it, my eyes were closed as instructed, and while I knew where I was and what was happening, I felt like I was too scared to open them. When Eugina was talking through my experience with me she asked me how I felt, all I was able to say was that I felt cold, confused and very uncomfortable. She asked if I could remember a time I had felt like this before. I couldn't tell her why I felt this or if I had before when it was. She then asked me if I did know, would I say? To which I would have done, I just didn't know why I was not comfortable with it. That night I couldn't sleep, so I thought I may as well use the time to see if I could better understand myself and what had happened that evening. As I went back through my life analysing many events and days to see where I had felt cold and confused before, I went back thirteen years before I found anything. I went back to that night out I had with Andy before going to Australia. The realisation was overwhelming, and I spent the rest of the night crying and feeling like a worthless piece of shit that no-one cared about. I thought about driving home that night as it felt easier to run away than to say anything to Eugina

133

that I had a new understanding. I was scared that I would be judged if I shared it and I couldn't sleep at all after that.

In the morning, I put on my sunglasses so that no-one could tell straight away that I'd been crying, as I tried to be what I was taught a man was. I saw Luke and he asked how I was doing. I explained that I had learnt something the night before and thought it best to share with him first before anyone else. He said that was great and that we'd all benefit from it and we'd go through it after breakfast. Something inside of me in that moment went, *"Oh fuck I need to get out of here."* Coaching had taught me that burying pain and emotions didn't help me in the long-term, so I resolved that I had to see this through even though I was scared to death.

After breakfast with the whole group together, Luke said to everyone that I had some realisations to share with everyone. My heart rate soared faster than Concorde, as I spoke about my sleepless night and tears the night before. Eugina encouraged me to tell the group more. I looked down at the table and hid my face in shame as I started to tell the story of going out with my mate and how I wound up staying at a flat overnight with one of the bar's regular customers. I remembered when we had got to his place that we chatted on the couch for a while and he had insisted that he opened my bottle of bubbly and both of us had a glass, yet mine was fizzing much more than his Champagne. Then I had fallen asleep or had passed out on his couch fully clothed but when I had woken up, I was laying naked on his bed and he was trying to penetrate me. By this time, I was balling like a baby in front of the group, feeling very fearful that they would think I was gay or no longer a man or just not strong enough. Luke then took me through a spiritual healing process. I don't remember all of it but a big part was of cutting the cord that tied us together in the spiritual realm and connected us at our knees. As the process came to an end, I noticed that every person there was also crying their eyes out, even the other guys and all of them had queued up to give me a hug.

After that day, the knee pain I had experienced for a long time and had put down to kneeling on cold workshop floors for years had gone. I didn't notice it at all, not even when I was back at work but what I did notice as I was working away from home, was that when I was away, I felt good, yet when I went home and through my doorway, my energy just went, so after a few weeks of this, I decided it was time to sell my house. I also felt ready to open myself to a special lady should one come my way.

26

Coming To America

In the same personal development singles group that I met the Norwegian nurse, a lady posted to share that she was embarking on a dating challenge; a date a week for a year until she met her man. I said it was a shame that there was an ocean between us, or I would be taking her out. We kept chatting and then she mentioned that she was going on a vacation to Ireland and I saw that as an opportunity to meet her. I found somewhere to stay, organised a hire car, went overseas and we spent three days together. We got on well and had a lot of fun, I literally swept her off of her feet dancing. Despite how good it felt between us, she decided that she wasn't ready for a relationship and had called off her challenge.

Initially, it triggered the old feelings of not being good enough, though as I caught it happening at the time with my new awareness, I was able to re-frame them quickly. Remembering that interview with James Hetfield, I wondered if I could write another song or two, though they turned out to be more like poems, they helped me to voice what was going on inside of me.

The kingdom of the heart.

In the begging I said I seek my queen,
My one in the world I've not yet seen,
To create our kingdom with a brand new start,
Yet, I forgot to mention it will be a kingdom of the heart,
No oceans, no customs, boundaries or wall,
Where every day in love we fall,
The day we met, my heart did melt,
Emotions inside still new not before I'd felt,
You tried to push away,

Yet here with you I choose to stay,
Sometimes, things may feel a little shit,
Your friend zone I refuse to fit,
 I can be a friend and play the rules as the law,
With intimacy, love and open heart, I'm so much more,
Not every day your body I can embrace,
Yet here I am holding your space,
For a little ribbon, countless men will die,
And so much more to be a hero in his lady's eye,
Some plans there may be on which life does piss,
With all my soul I know that I got this!
With the appreciation and praise that you show,
My masculine energy sure does grow,
Do I find you sexy as you feel your body's a mess,
No doubt in me oh fuck yes!!
My twins in a dream brought you to me,
Yet the reason you have yet to see,
No success is needed to earn love you see,
Just in your beautiful heart you must be,
As other men never saw the goddess in you,
With my heart and soul I feel I truly do,
We know not where this will go,
In our creator we choose to trust and its flow,
When I'm in my heart or drop to my head,
You're the one I desire to take to bed,
We may be a world apart
Yet still together in the kingdom of the heart.

Not long after and out of the blue, I connected with another lady in America. We chatted and had video calls for a while, talking very deeply, sharing deep beliefs and experiences and the things that had challenged us to grow over the years. The first video call we got to have, I felt like I could share my deepest darkest secrets with her and be fully safe to do so, and several times I did so. There was something in me that said you have to meet her whatever it takes. Somehow, I found the money to book the flights I needed. She was looking forward to meeting me and getting to know me on much deeper levels as I was with her. I only had a week free to travel there, stay for a few days and return home. I asked if she could recommend somewhere close by to stay as I didn't want to just assume she would put me up. She said staying with her was not a problem but if I were uncomfortable, I could stay elsewhere, or she would make up the spare room. As long as I had somewhere to sleep, I'd be happy. We both shared similar visions of how we wanted a relationship to be.

In most cases. the depth of this conversation wouldn't happen before meeting in person but with us living in separate countries and my having children meant that I couldn't emigrate to another country and wouldn't leave them. We had to talk about the important things upfront to be more certain that it could go somewhere if we liked each other after physically meeting. She lived with her dog and two cats. I often imagined her being like a real-life Snow White, surrounded by animals to care for and nurture. Both of us believed that the connection we had was amazing and had very high hopes for us having a future together.

The day of travel came, and she messaged me to say that she had made up the spare room before I'd even left England. By the time I landed in America to catch my internal flight to her city, she messaged me to say that she had taken her dog to be put to sleep at the vets and was feeling a little emotional. I let her know that I was sure I could handle her however she was feeling. She met me at the airport, and it was incredible to actually be face to face, we hugged and kissed. As the week progressed, we had a few deep talks, although I felt like I was talking to a different person than the one I'd spoken to so many times online. Most of the times that I tried to get closer to her either mentally, emotionally, or physically, I would be pushed away. I didn't feel at all welcome and I couldn't understand what was going on. I knew that she was texting her friends about me the whole time, but I could only imagine what about. As I knew that she had a lot going on emotionally with her dog, I didn't want to burden her further with my confused feelings and uncertainty. Being in another country, sharing a house with someone emotional who had a gun, made me feel very vulnerable, almost as if I had to walk on eggshells to not say or do the wrong thing. It was very challenging. The last night I was there, she let me know how she felt after feeling triggered by me placing a hand on her shoulder when she said a piece of music made her feel bad.

In her book, *"The Queen's Code,"* Alison Armstrong talks about women having a sword of emasculation; this felt more like a lightsaber. It cut and cauterized at the same time. Her words were deeply personal and hurt as if many of my fears and vulnerabilities I had shared with her over the time we had been talking were now being used against me. I felt like Luke Skywalker when he was told Darth Vader was his father and he chose to fall instead of turn to the Dark Side.

I didn't sleep a wink that night, even though I knew we were getting up early to go and see the sunrise before she took me to the airport to head home. Where had the lady I had been talking to before disappeared to? Where she would openly express how she felt and I could understand what she was going through when we chatted online, whilst I was there, I couldn't get through. It was like she was closed off to me and I couldn't work out why. A great many questions buzzed around in my mind as I attempted to get some sleep.

When she dropped me off at the airport, I asked if she wanted another kiss, she said yes, I thought it a little bizarre that she now wanted to kiss the man she had been pushing away all week. I wanted to know if she was actually interested in me and if she was, how much. I replied, *"Well, you have been telling me to let you come to me this week, so here is your chance - if you want that kiss, come to England and get it."*

27

Understanding Emotions (Or Not)

We messaged each other a few times once I was back home, so we could both learn and grow from the experience and it took a few weeks to dig down through some of the stuff, for me especially. It turned out that even though we had both been communicating deeply and honestly, we both had bits that we had miscommunicated and misunderstood. With some parts, they turned out to be made up stories we'd created in our heads as to what things meant, which in reality were way off. We still message each other and chat from time to time but nowhere near as often or as deeply as we once did. There were things that both of us did that reminded each other of painful relationships in our pasts, triggering fight or flight responses which made any communication very difficult and skewed.

After a few days of being home, I reached out to a few trusted friends, one of which being the Norwegian Nurse, as I needed a perspective from someone else who knew me deeply. I shared my experience with her and then she asked me a question I wasn't expecting. She asked if I had told her I was Asperger's or on the Autism spectrum. My idea of Autism and Asperger's was, I have found, to be completely incorrect, but it was people who got overwhelmed easily by sounds and had to wear earphones to protect them or shake their arms about a lot, I knew I didn't do any of that. Wanting to understand myself I started looking into it. I was also made aware of Childhood Emotional Neglect (CEN) at the same time, which comes from children not being taught about emotions when they're growing up. I couldn't remember feelings or emotions being talked about which I wondered if this were a possibility too.

While watching the Hulk and the Avengers with my children after returning home, as I saw Bruce Banner trying to keep hulk inside and not get angry, I saw myself in a new light. Hulk was part of Bruce, a big part that many people misunderstood and hated because others hated him as he hurt people, Bruce learned to hate him too. My dark side made up of my anger, my frustration, my fear, my sadness, my loneliness, and all are parts of me that I had been trying to hide from everyone as I believed that anyone who saw those parts of me they wouldn't like or love and it was all intertwined into one big mess. The more I hid and suppressed those parts of me, the more powerful they became and the less control I had over them. They were all me, different times, different ages and events, but all me and all part of me. Some spiritual people may call this my inner child. My inner child or my hulk didn't want to be pushed away, squashed down and hidden, much the same as my own children. He needed to be seen, felt, heard, appreciated, accepted, and loved; by me, myself and I.

I am still looking within myself and researching what is possible for me in terms of being aware of and understanding my own feelings in the present moment. It is still very much as said in the personal development world, a work in progress.

28

Running Wild And Running Free

Learning to love myself after thirty years of not doing so has not been and is not an easy process. It certainly doesn't happen in a heartbeat or overnight. I could write a book on that part of the journey alone and maybe in the future, I will.

I sold my house in June 2019, having explored many options of where and how to live and had many people tell me what they believed I should do. I decided to do what I believed to be right for me and I have had no regrets. I chose against buying another house, not that I would have been in a position to do so after settling all of the divorce debts. I looked at renting another house only to find it would have cost me almost double the cost of my mortgage for a smaller house.

For me, it made no sense to work all hours for money to live in a four-walled and ceiling box that I would never own and never see because I'd be at work a lot of the time. I would always have the worry about what would happen if I lost my income stream, which would prevent me from being able to relax or be fully present with my family or friends. Instead, I bought the biggest van I could find that was in good condition and used my mechanical skills to convert it into a mobile home. I'm almost debt-free and aim to be by the end of the year. I am mortgage-free and almost rent-free, except for a few campsite fees. I am free to work anywhere I like, providing that I can be at home at the weekends to be with my kids, or at least pick them up for a weekend adventure.

I am the most at peace I have been with myself, my life and my family that I have ever been. My life is no longer controlled or destined by other people's opinions, beliefs of me and what I *"should"* be or how I *"ought"* to live. I am no longer controlled or subscribe to the, *"Get a good job, work hard, buy a house, have a family, try to save money and become mortgage free by sixty and retire on less than you earned before, with an exhausted body to live with,"* society idea. That makes me feel like I'm boxed in a box that I don't fit in - like a prison with an illusion of freedom to me.

For many of the years described in this book I have felt like I was in captivity, a bit like a tiger that should be roaming out in the jungle or desert, they should be out running wild and running free, not in a zoo with a fraction of what is possible.

The difficulties that I experienced with not feeling wholly connected to my emotions or of what they really were hampered my life and particularly relationships, as you'll have grasped from my story. Every part of my personal development inspired me to better understand myself and what made me tick and how that impacted upon my life with others. The benefit I found within coaching and the shifts I was able to make were so great that I knew my purpose was to help others to create and experience better relationships through the coaching business that I set up.

If you resonate with any of my experiences and are looking for support and to make changes in personal relationships then I invite you to reach out to me via the contact methods on the following page.

Contact Page

You can connect with me here:
www.facebook.com/OfficialLoveEngineer/
Email: runwild-runfree@love-engineers.win

And if you wish to work with me one on one or learn more about my signature Relationship Coaching Programme *"Love Engineering 2020"* or wish to book me for speaking opportunities please reach out to me through one of these channels.